Stahl's Illustrated

Antidepressants

Stephen M. Stahl
University of California at San Diego

Nancy Muntner
Illustrations

Angela Felker
Editor

CAMBRIDGE
UNIVERSITY PRESS

CAMBRIDGE
UNIVERSITY PRESS

University Printing House, Cambridge CB2 8BS, United Kingdom

One Liberty Plaza, 20th Floor, New York, NY 10006, USA

477 Williamstown Road, Port Melbourne, VIC 3207, Australia

314–321, 3rd Floor, Plot 3, Splendor Forum, Jasola District Centre, New Delhi – 110025, India

79 Anson Road, #06–04/06, Singapore 079906

Cambridge University Press is part of the University of Cambridge.

It furthers the University's mission by disseminating knowledge in the pursuit of education, learning and research at the highest international levels of excellence.

www.cambridge.org
Information on this title: www.cambridge.org/9780521758529

First published 2009
3rd printing 2018

Printed and bound in Great Britain by Clays Ltd, Elcograf S.p.A.

A catalogue record for this publication is available from the British Library

Library of Congress Cataloging in Publication Data

Stahl, S. M.
Antidepressants / Stephen M. Stahl.
p. ; cm. - (Stahl's illustrated series)
Approved for a maximum of 3.0 AMA PRA Category 1 credits.
Includes bibliographical references and index.
ISBN 978-0-521-75852-9 (pbk.)
1. Antidepresssants. I. Title. II. Series: Stahl's illustrated series.
[DNLM: 1. Antidespressive Agents-pharmacology. 2. Depressive Disorder-drug therapy. QV 77.5 S781a 2009]
RM332.S727 2009
615'.78-dc22

2008054879

ISBN 978-0-521-75852-9 paperback

PREFACE

These books are designed to be fun. All concepts are illustrated by full-color images. The text can be used as a supplement to figures, images, and tables. The visual learner will find that this book makes psychopharmacology concepts easy to master, while the non-visual learner may enjoy a shortened text version of complex psychopharmacology concepts. Each chapter builds upon previous chapters, synthesizing information from basic biology and diagnostics to building treatment plans and dealing with complications and comorbidities.

Novices may want to approach this Pocketbook by first looking through all the graphics, gaining a feel for the visual vocabulary on which our psychopharmacology concepts rely. After this once-over glance, we suggest going back through the book to incorporate the images with text from figure legends. Learning from visual concepts and textual supplements should reinforce one another, providing you with solid conceptual understanding at each step along the way.

Readers more familiar with these topics should find that going back and forth between images and text provides an interaction with which to vividly conceptualize complex psychopharmacology. You may find yourself using this book frequently to refresh your psychopharmacological knowledge. You may also find yourself referring your colleagues to this desk reference.

This Pocketbook is intended as a conceptual overview of different topics; we provide you with a visual-based language to incorporate the rules of psychopharmacology at the sacrifice of discussing the exceptions to these rules. A Suggested Readings section at the end of this Pocketbook gives you a good start for more in-depth learning about particular concepts presented here.

When you come across an abbreviation or figure you don't understand, you can refer to the Abbreviation and Symbols legend in the back. After referring to these several times you will begin to develop proficiency in the visual vocabulary of psychopharmacology. Stahl's Essential Psychopharmacology, 3rd Edition, and Stahl's Essential Psychopharmacology: The Prescriber's Guide, 2nd Edition can be helpful supplementary tools for more in-depth information on particular topics in this Pocketbook. Now you can also search topics in psychopharmacology on the Neuroscience Education Institute's website (www.neiglobal.com) for lectures, courses, slides and related articles.

Whether you are a novice or an experienced psychopharmacologist, hopefully this book will lead you to think critically about the complexities involved in psychiatric disorders and their treatments.

Best wishes for your educational journey into the fascinating field of psychopharmacology!

Stephen M. Stahl

Table of Contents

CME Information

CME credit has expired for this activity (2/28/15). You are welcome and encouraged to complete the activity and posttest for your personal enrichment, but will not be able to receive credit nor print a certificate for this activity.

(Original CME Information)

Overview

This book aims to visually explain the concepts behind the neurobiology of depression, as well as the current and novel treatment options available to clinicians to treat depression. The book is divided into eight chapters for ease of reading and referencing. Chapter 1 focuses on the neurobiology behind depression, with an emphasis on the neurotransmitters involved in the experience of depressive symptomatology: serotonin, norepinephrine and dopamine. Chapter 2 begins the introduction of antidepressant drug classes, with an overview and in-depth explanation of each drug in the SSRI and SNRI classes. Chapter 3 covers NDRIs and NRIs; Chapter 4 features SNDIs and SARIs; Chapter 5 examines the older generation of antidepressants— MAOIs and TCAs; and Chapter 6 introduces novel treatment options for managing depression. Chapter 7 focuses on depression in women, emphasizing the role that estrogen plays in the experience of depressive symptomatology. Chapter 8 reviews the pharmacokinetics of antidepressants, and introduces algorithms commonly used to treat depression. The visual component of this book is designed to allow the reader to easily grasp complex concepts.

Target Audience

This activity has been developed for prescribers specializing in psychiatry. There are no prerequisites. All other health care providers interested in psychopharmacology, are welcome for advanced study.

Statement of Need

The following unmet needs and professional practice gaps regarding antidepressants were revealed following a critical analysis of activity feedback, expert faculty assessment, literature review, and through new medical knowledge:

- Not all antidepressants are efficacious in all patients; thus, it is important for mental health professionals to be aware of alternative options.
- Full remission and recovery is still the gold standard for depression, yet only 50% of responders actually achieve remission.
- The most common residual symptoms of treatments for depression are insomnia, hypersomnia and physical fatigue/pain, and executive dysfunction.

To help address clinician performance deficits with respect to treating depression, quality improvement efforts need to provide education that will increase understanding of the neurobiology of psychiatric disease states and the pharmacology of available, new, and in-development medications.

Learning Objectives

After completing this activity, participants should be better able to:

- Recognize the symptoms and circuits of depression and how to treat them in clinical practice
- Understand the pharmacology of antidepressants
- Describe the pharmacodynamics and pharmacokinetics of antidepressants
- Discuss how to select and combine antidepressant treatments
- Highlight new drugs in development for the treatment of depression

Accreditation and Credit Designation Statements

The Neuroscience Education Institute is accredited by the Accreditation Council for Continuing Medical Education to provide continuing medical education for physicians.

The Neuroscience Education Institute designates this enduring material for a maxi¬mum of 3.0 *AMA PRA Category 1 Credits*™. Physicians should claim only the credit commensurate with the extent of their participation in the activity.

Nurses: for all of your CNE requirements for recertification, the ANCC will accept *AMA PRA Category 1 Credits*™ from organizations accredited by the ACCME.

Physician Assistants: the NCCPA accepts *AMA PRA Category 1 Credits*™ from organizations accredited by the AMA (providers accredited by the ACCME).

A certificate of participation for completing this activity will also be available.

Activity Instructions

This CME activity is in the form of a printed monograph and incorporates instructional design to enhance your retention of the information and pharmacological concepts that are being presented. You are advised to go through the figures in this activity from beginning to end, followed by the text, and then complete the posttest and activity evaluation. The estimated time for completion of this activity is 3.0 hours.

NEI Disclosure Policy

It is the policy of the Neuroscience Education Institute to ensure balance, independence, objectivity, and scientific rigor in all its educational activities. Therefore, all individuals in a position to influence or control content development are required by

NEI to disclose any financial relationships or apparent conflicts of interest. Although potential conflicts of interest are identified and resolved prior to the activity being presented, it remains for the participant to determine whether outside interests reflect a possible bias in either the exposition or the conclusions presented.

These materials have been peer-reviewed to ensure the scientific accuracy and medical relevance of information presented and its independence from commercial bias. The Neuroscience Education Institute takes responsibility for the content, quality, and scientific integrity of this CME activity.

Individual Disclosure Statements

Author

Stephen M. Stahl, MD, PhD
Adjunct Professor, Department of Psychiatry, University of California, San Diego School of Medicine
Honorary Visiting Senior Fellow, University of Cambridge, UK
Grant/Research: AstraZeneca, BioMarin, Dainippon Sumitomo, Forest, Genomind, Lilly, Merck, Pamlab, Pfizer, PGxHealth/Trovis, Schering-Plough, Sepracor, Servier, Shire, Torrent
Consultant/Advisor: Abbott, Advent, Alkermes, Arena, AstraZeneca, BioMarin, Boehringer Ingelheim, Bristol-Myers Squibb, Cypress, Dainippon Sumitomo, Forest, Genomind, Janssen, Division of Ortho-McNeil-Janssen, Jazz, Labopharm, Lilly, Lundbeck, Merck, Neuronetics, Novartis, Ono, Orexigen, Otsuka America, Pamlab, Pfizer, PGxHealth/Clinical Data, Rexahn, Royalty, Schering-Plough, Servier, Shire, Valeant, VIVUS
Speakers Bureau: Dainippon Sumitomo, Lilly, Merck, Pamlab, Sepracor, Sunovion

Content Editors

Angela Felker, MA
Associate Medical Writer, Neuroscience Education Institute, Carlsbad, CA
No financial relationships to disclose.

Meghan Grady
Director, Content Development, Neuroscience Education Institute, Carlsbad, CA
No financial relationships to disclose.

Peer Reviewers

(for original release)
Scott A. Irwin, MD, PhD
Director, Psychiatry Programs, The Institute for Palliative Medicine, at San Diego Hospice, San Diego, CA
No financial relationships to disclose.

(for rerelease)
Steven S. Simring, MD, MPH
Clinical Associate Professor, Department of Psychiatry, Columbia University College of Physicians and Surgeons, New York State Psychiatric Institute, New York City
No financial relationships to disclose.

Design Staff

Nancy Muntner
Director, Medical Illustrations, Neuroscience Education Institute, Carlsbad, CA
No financial relationships to disclose.

Disclosed financial relationships with conflicts of interest have been reviewed by the Neuroscience Education Institute CME Advisory Board Chair and resolved. All faculty and planning committee members have attested that their financial relationships do not affect their ability to present well-balanced, evidence-based content for this activity.

Disclosure of Off-Label Use

This educational activity may include discussion of unlabeled and/or investigational uses of agents that are not currently labeled for such use by the FDA. Please consult the product prescribing information for full disclosure of labeled uses.

Disclaimer

Participants have an implied responsibility to use the newly acquired information from this activity to enhance patient outcomes and their own professional development. The information presented in this educational activity is not meant to serve as a guideline for patient management. Any procedures, medications, or other courses of diagnosis or treatment discussed or suggested in this educational activity should not be used by clinicians without evaluation of their patients' conditions and possible contraindications or dangers in use, review of any applicable manufacturer's product information, and comparison with recommendations of other authorities. Primary references and full prescribing information should be consulted.

Sponsorship Information

This activity is sponsored by the Neuroscience Education Institute.

Support

This activity is supported solely by the sponsor, Neuroscience Education Institute. Neither the Neuroscience Education Institute nor Stephen M. Stahl, MD, PhD, has received any funds or grants in support of this educational activity.

Objectives

- Recognize the symptoms and circuits of depression and how to treat them in clinical practice
- Understand the pharmacology of antidepressants
- Describe the pharmacodynamics and pharmacokinetics of antidepressants
- Discuss how to select and combine antidepressant treatments
- Highlight new drugs in development for the treatment of depression

Stahl's Illustrated

Chapter 1

Neurobiology of Depression

Depression can affect every aspect of life. A patient undergoing a major depressive episode who receives treatment with any antidepressant will often experience symptomatic improvement. However, oftentimes treatment does not reach the goal of remission (complete cessation of all symptoms of depression) until several different pharmacotherapies have been utilized, possibly in combination. Understanding the neurobiology underlying depressive symptomatology may allow clinicians the opportunity to treat the symptoms specifically, based upon brain mechanisms and the interplay among genes, circuits and symptoms. This chapter focuses on the neurobiology of depression, and offers a review of the three monoamines hypothetically linked not only to the symptoms of a major depressive episode, but also to the treatment of those symptoms.

Mood Chart

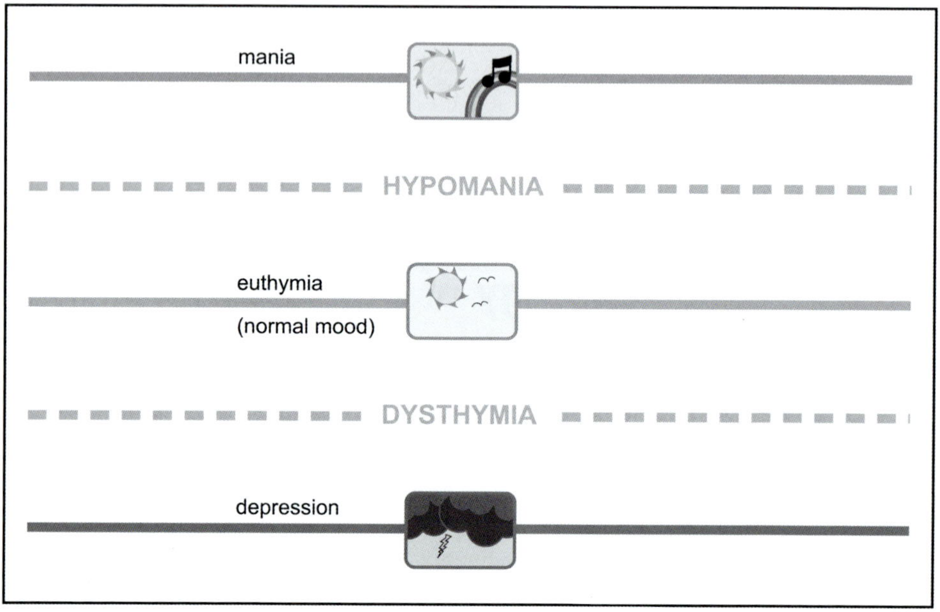

FIGURE 1.1. Mood charts illustrate a spectrum of syndromal states upon which a patient's mood can be charted over time. Mood monitoring can be conducted intermittently in a clinical setting or continuously via patient self-report in the form of a mood diary. Tracking the course of illness can greatly assist in identifying disease states, diagnosing accurately, and assessing treatment response.

Depressive Temperament and Dysthymia

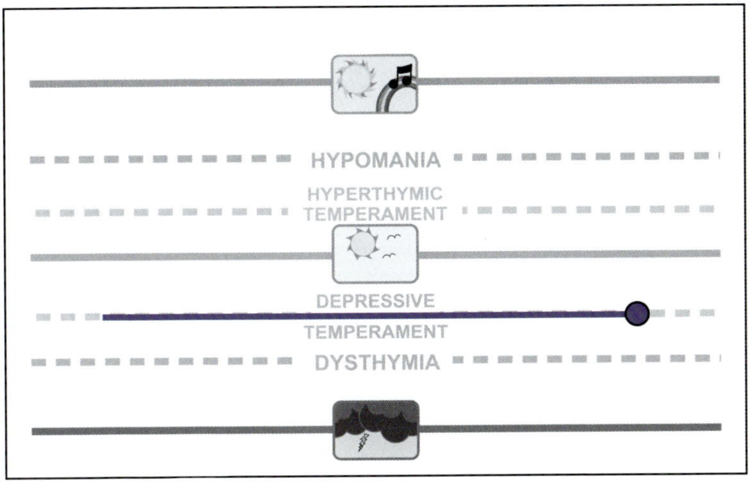

FIGURE 1.2. Patients with a depressive temperament may be regularly sad or apathetic but do not have a sufficient degree or number of symptoms to qualify for the diagnosis of dysthymia or a major depressive episode. Individuals with depressive temperament may be more at risk for a future mood disorder.

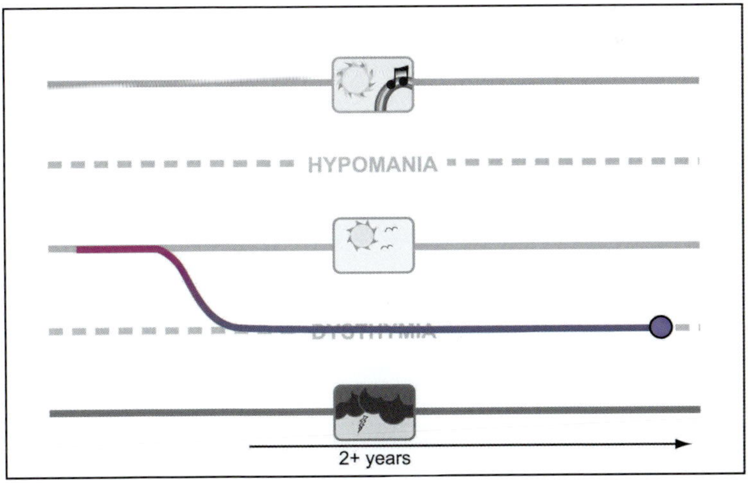

FIGURE 1.3. Dysthymia is a less severe form of depression than major depressive disorder (MDD), but is long-lasting and generally unrelenting for two years or more.

Identifying Mood Disorders:
Depression and Double Depression

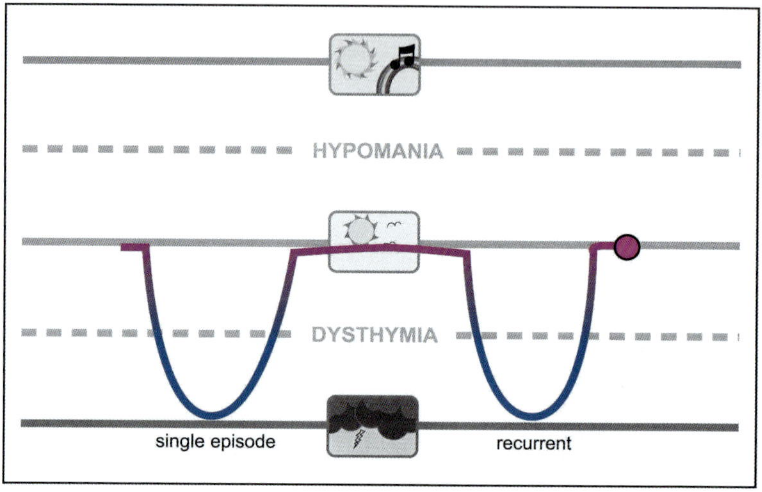

FIGURE 1.4. Major depressive disorder (MDD) is characterized by single or recurrent major depressive episode(s); most people with MDD will experience recurrent episodes. This is the most common mood disorder.

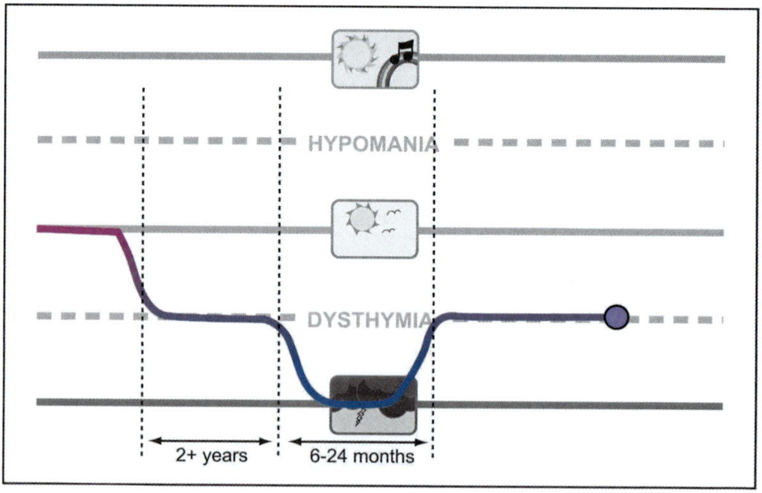

FIGURE 1.5. Double depression is characterized by unremitting dysthymia interrupted by major depressive episode(s). Between episodes there is poor inter-episode recovery.

Unipolar vs. Bipolar Depression

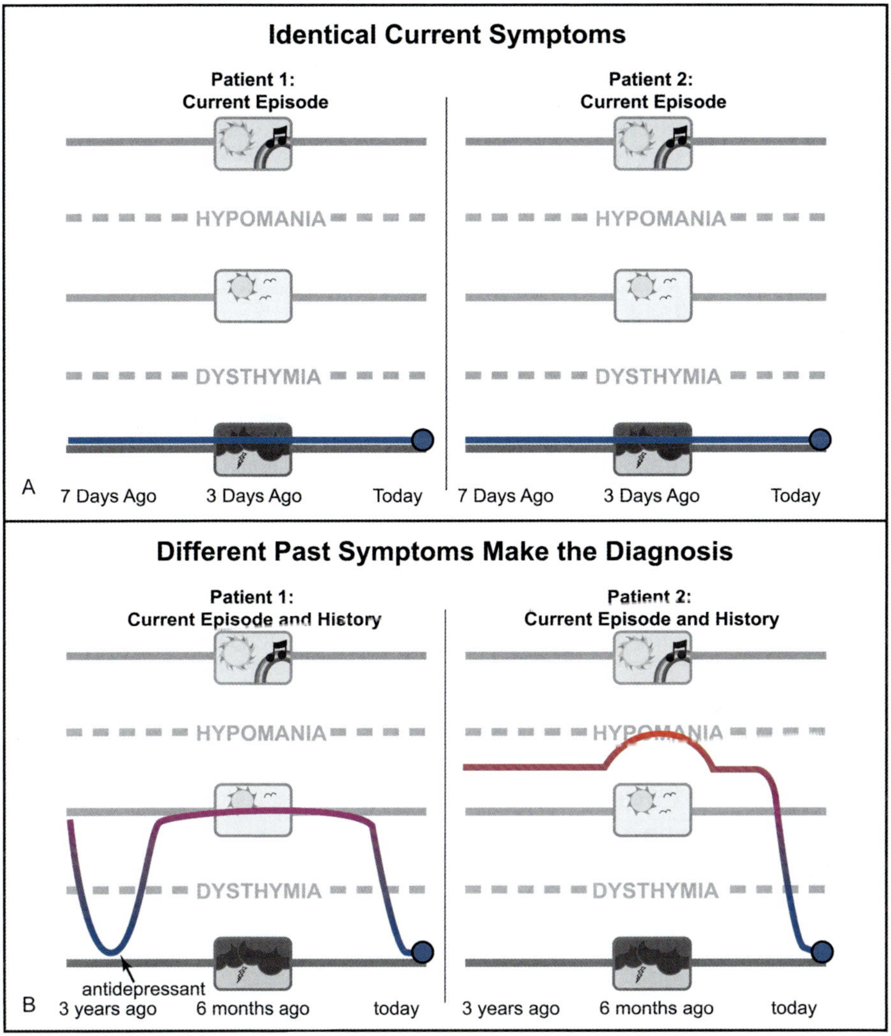

FIGURE 1.6. Although both patients in this mood chart are presenting with identical current symptoms of a major depressive episode over the past several days (A), patient 1 has unipolar depression whereas patient 2 has bipolar depression. So, what is the difference? The pattern of past symptoms (B) is quite different; for example, patient 1 has experienced a prior depressive episode whereas patient 2 has experienced a prior hypomanic episode.

Are Mood Disorders Progressive?

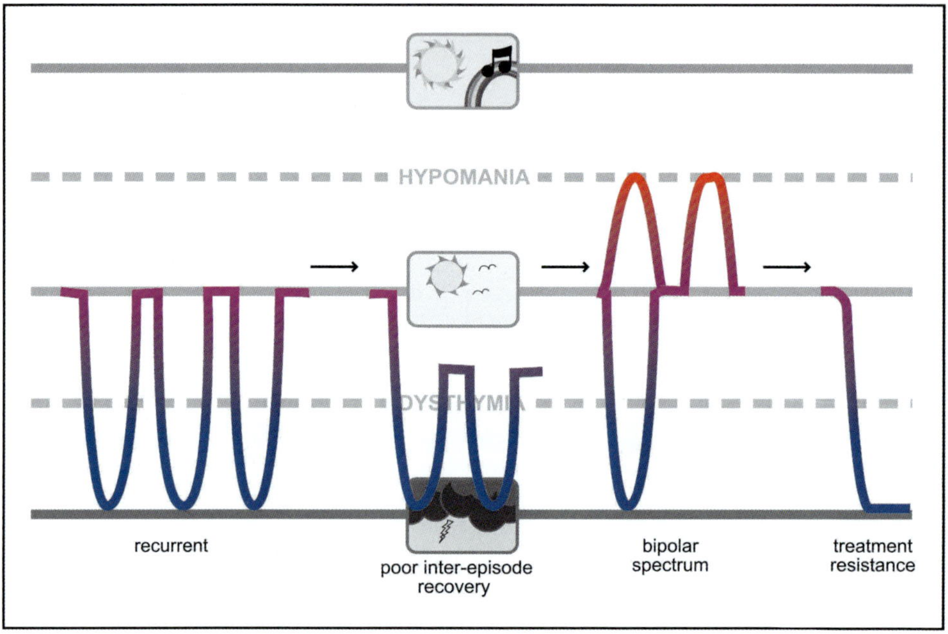

FIGURE 1.7. Is major depressive disorder (MDD) progressive? Some believe that un(der)treated unipolar depression can develop into a bipolar spectrum condition, eventually to the point of treatment resistance.

Common Comorbidities in Major Depressive Disorder (MDD)

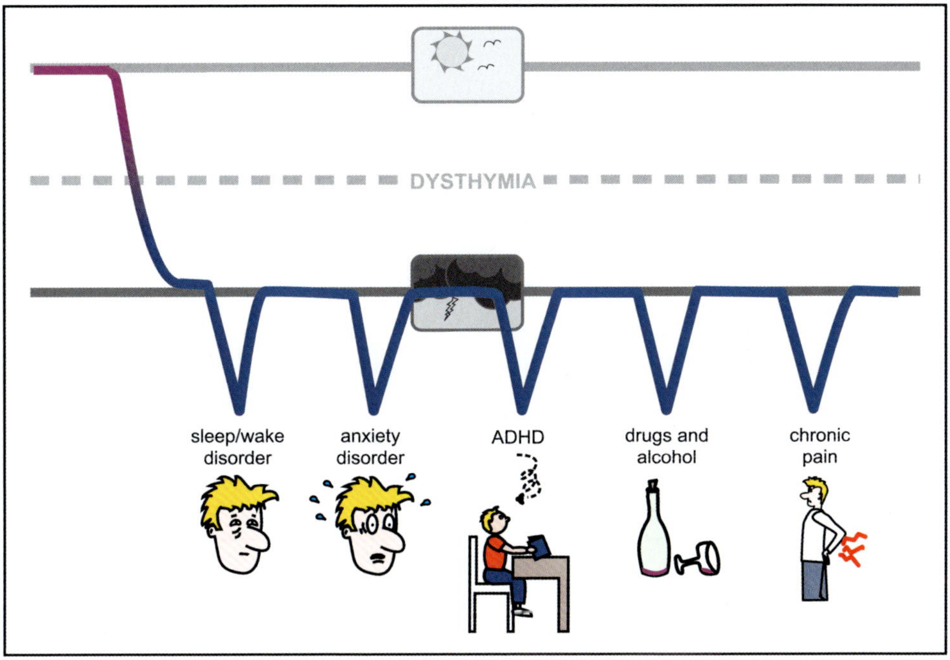

FIGURE 1.8. Some common comorbidities in major depressive disorder (MDD) include sleep/wake problems, anxiety, attention deficit hyperactivity disorder (ADHD), substance abuse and chronic pain.

Monoamine Hypothesis of Depression

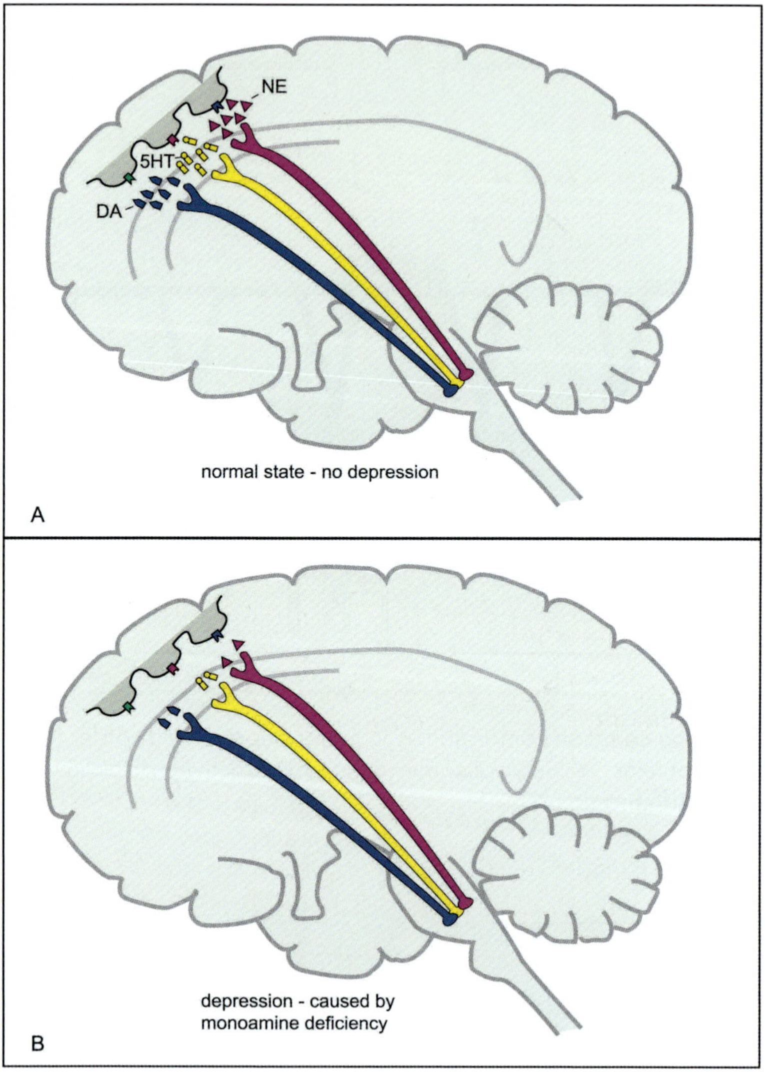

FIGURE 1.9. There are three key monoamines: dopamine (DA), norepinephrine (NE) and serotonin (5-hydroxytryptamine or 5HT) (A). The classical "monoamine hypothesis of depression" states that depression results from a deficiency in one or more of these three monoamines (B).

Monoamine Hypothesis of Antidepressant Action

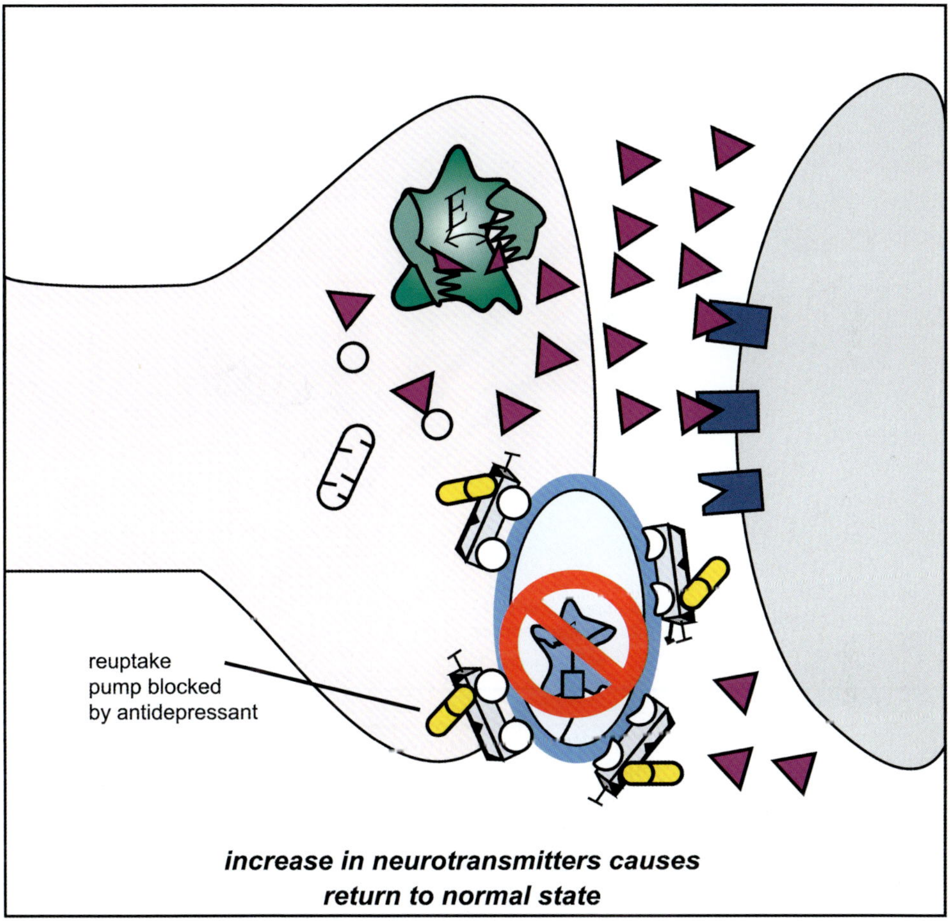

FIGURE 1.10. According to this hypothesis, depression caused by deficiency of 5HT, NE and/or DA is theoretically returned to a normal state by antidepressants that increase the synaptic action of monoamines, such as those that block presynaptic monoamine transporters (also called reuptake pumps) as shown here.

Monoamine Receptor Hypothesis of Depression

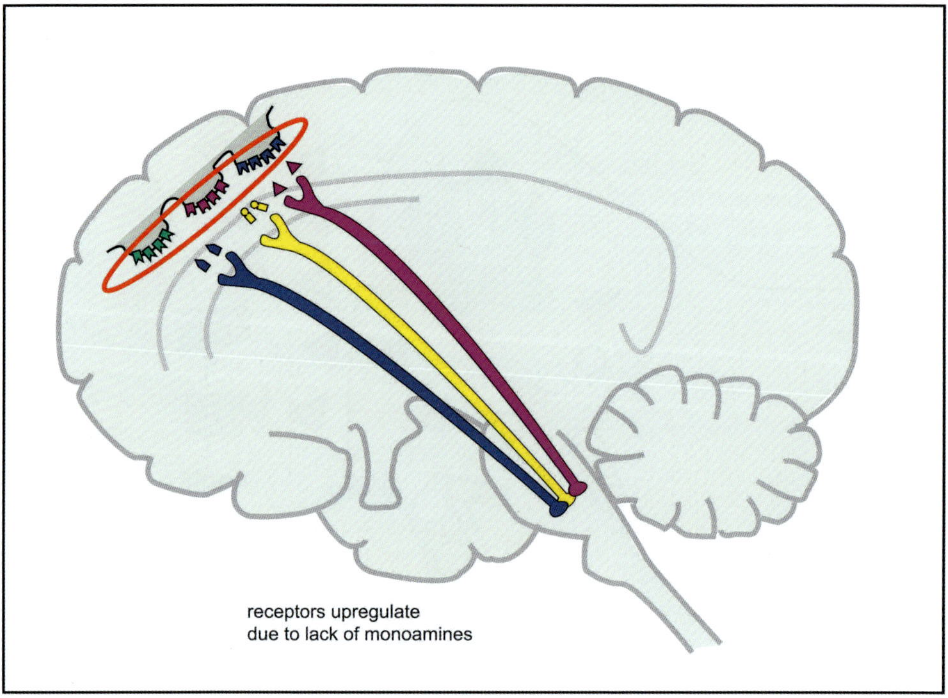

FIGURE 1.11. The monoamine receptor hypothesis builds on the classic monoamine hypothesis of depression by suggesting that decreased activity of monoamine neurotransmitters (5HT, NE, DA) causes upregulation of postsynaptic monoamine receptors, leading to depression.

Monoamine Receptor Hypothesis of Antidepressant Action

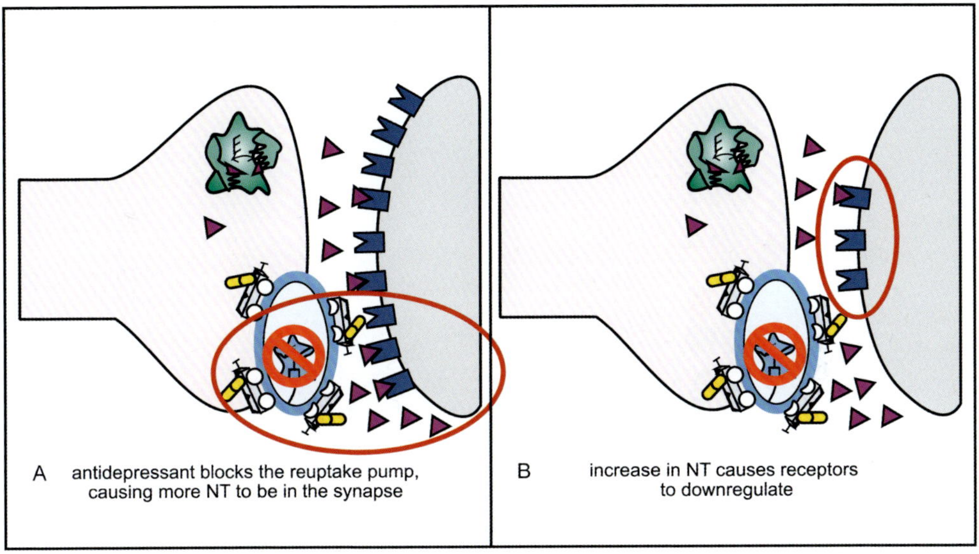

FIGURE 1.12. The monoamine receptor hypothesis suggests that if depression is caused by upregulation of monoamine receptors, antidepressants act by ultimately downregulating monoamine receptors over time. In frame A, an antidepressant acutely blocks the reuptake pump, allowing for more neurotransmitter in the synapse. Frame B indicates that chronically increased availability of neurotransmitter over time leads to downregulation of receptors. The time course for this to occur (several days to weeks) is consistent with both delayed onset of antidepressant effects and the time required to develop tolerance to side effects.

Monoamine Hypothesis of Antidepressant Action on Gene Expression

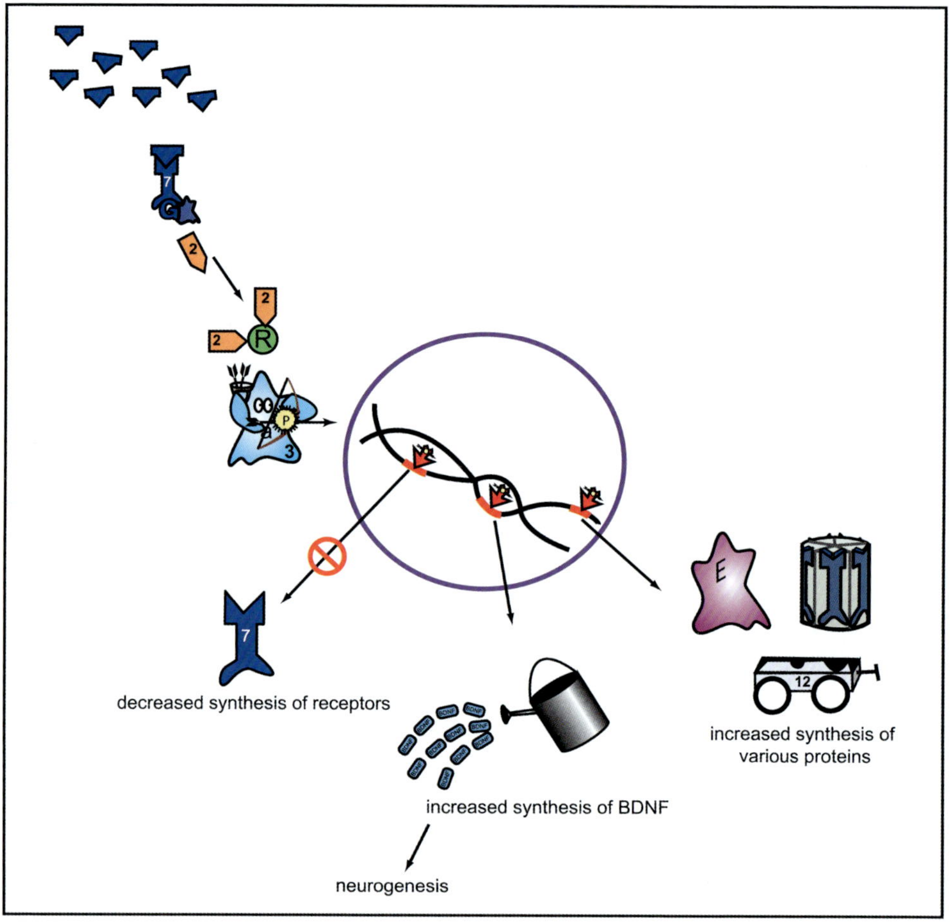

FIGURE 1.13. Based on the monoamine hypothesis of depression, antidepressant administration can theoretically create a return to a normal mood state by increasing the levels of monoamines. Here, the downstream consequences of increased monoamine production by antidepressants are shown. The neurotransmitter at the top is assumed to increase via antidepressant administration. The resulting cascade affects expression of critical genes, including downregulation or upregulation of various gene products, as depicted.

Time Course of Antidepressant Effects

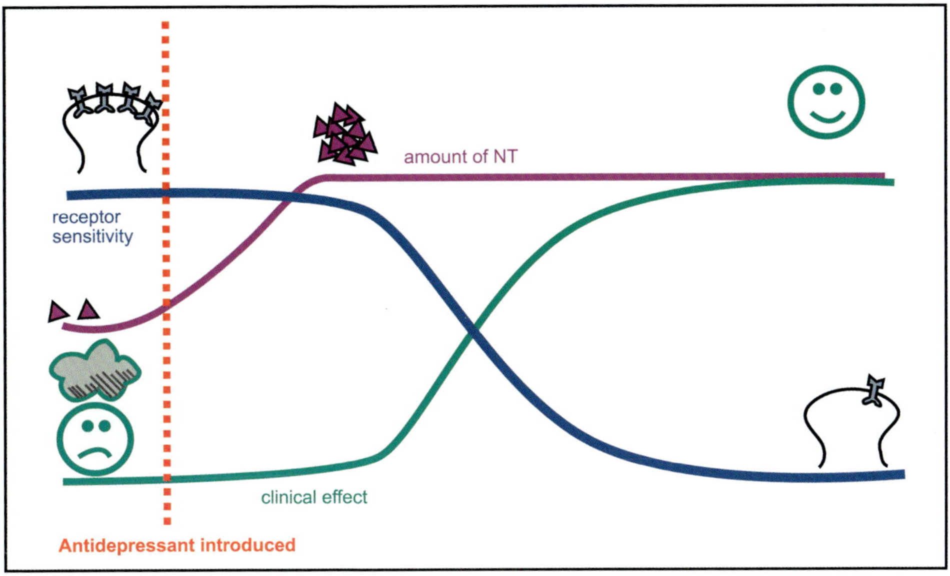

FIGURE 1.14. Antidepressant drugs have three time courses—clinical changes, neurotransmitter changes, and receptor sensitivity changes. While the neurotransmitter changes often occur rapidly after initial administration, clinical changes and receptor changes (i.e., downregulation) take longer to occur. This observation has resulted in the hypothesis that neurotransmitter receptor sensitivity may mediate the clinical changes seen after antidepressant administration, including the production of therapeutic antidepressant effects and the development of tolerance to side effects, all of which occur over a few weeks of time.

Synthesis and Metabolism of Serotonin

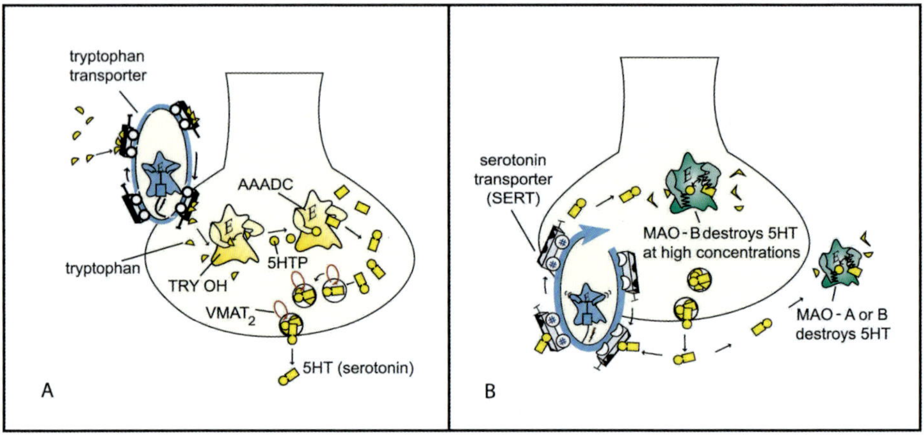

FIGURE 1.15. Serotonin (also known as 5-hydroxy-tryptamine or 5HT) is one of the three principal monoamines. It is synthesized from the amino acid tryptophan (TRY), which is transported into the serotonin neuron by the tryptophan transporter (A), a transporter that is distinct from the serotonin transporter shown in B. After tryptophan is pumped into the serotonin neuron, it is hydroxylated by the rate-limiting enzyme for 5HT synthesis, namely tryptophan hydroxylase or TRY-OH (A) to 5-hydroxy-tryptophan (5HTP). 5HTP is then decarboxylated to 5HT by the enzyme aromatic amino acid decarboxylase (AADC) (A). 5HT synthesized in the presynaptic neuron is then transported into synaptic vesicles via the synaptic vesicle pump VMAT2 (vesicular monoamine transporter 2) (A). There it is stored until released during neurotransmission (B).

5HT released into the synapse during neurotransmission is either transported back into the serotonin neuron or metabolized and destroyed extraneuronally by either MAO-A or MAO-B (B). If 5HT inside the neuron is not quickly transported into synaptic vesicles (A), it will be destroyed by MAO-B inside the neuron (B).

Serotonin Receptors: Part 1

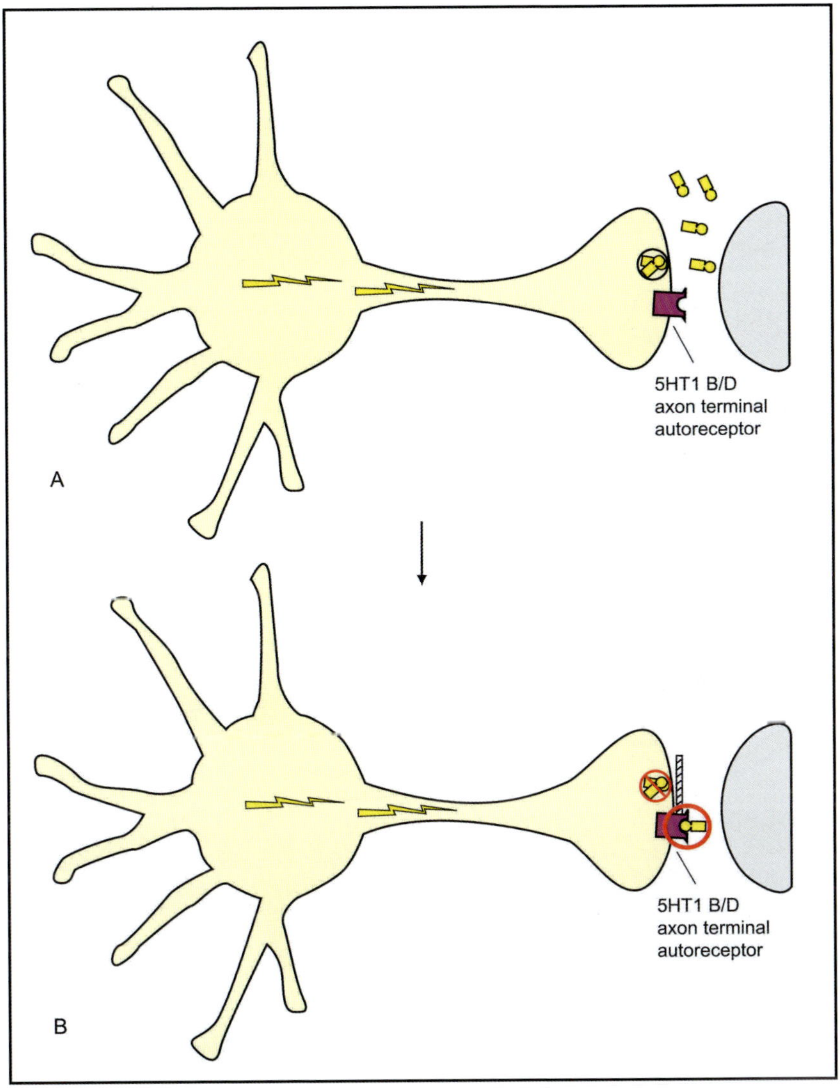

FIGURE 1.16. Presynaptic 5HT1B/D receptors are located on the axon terminal (A). These receptors inhibit further 5HT release when they detect the presence of 5HT in the synapse (B). This can happen when 5HT builds up in the synapse and is therefore available to the autoreceptor (B).

Serotonin Receptors: Part 2

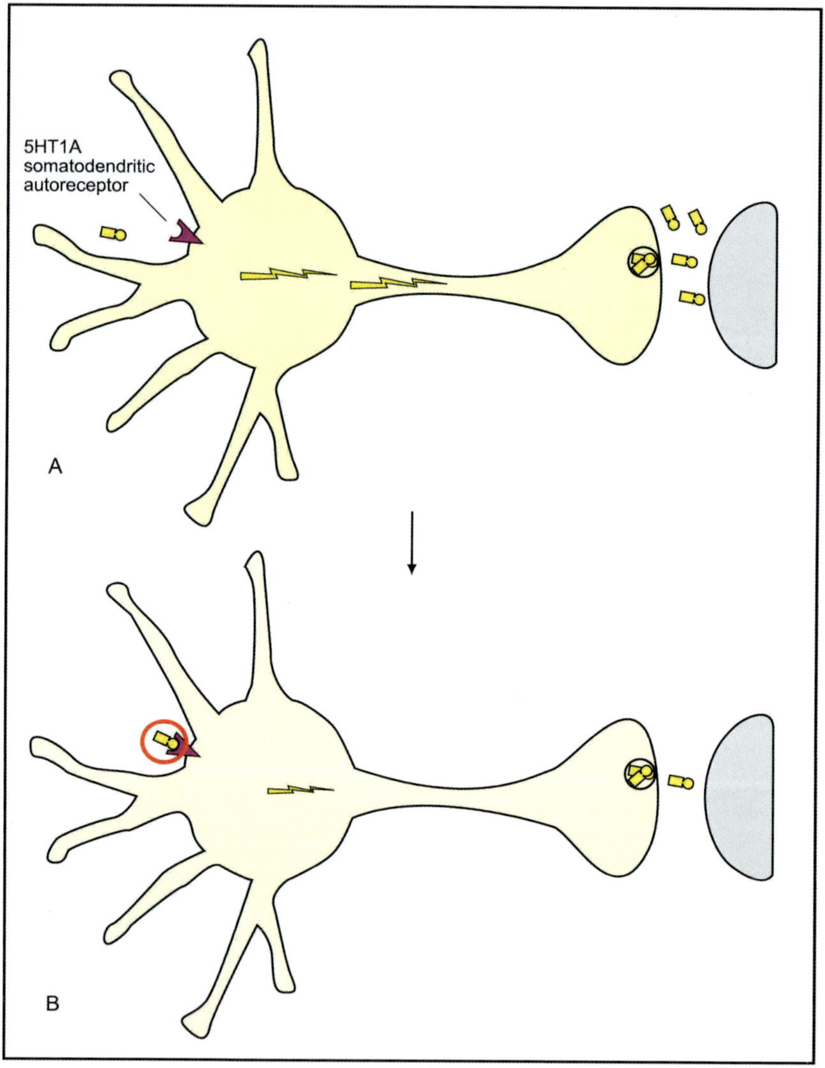

FIGURE 1.17. Presynaptic 5HT1A receptors are located on the cell body and dendrites, thus termed somatodendritic autoreceptors (A). These receptors shut down 5HT impulse flow when 5HT binds to them (B). When serotonin binds to the somatodendritic receptor (top), it reduces neuronal electrical activity shown in the neuron, and decreases the amount of serotonin shown in the synapse (bottom).

Serotonin Receptors: Part 3

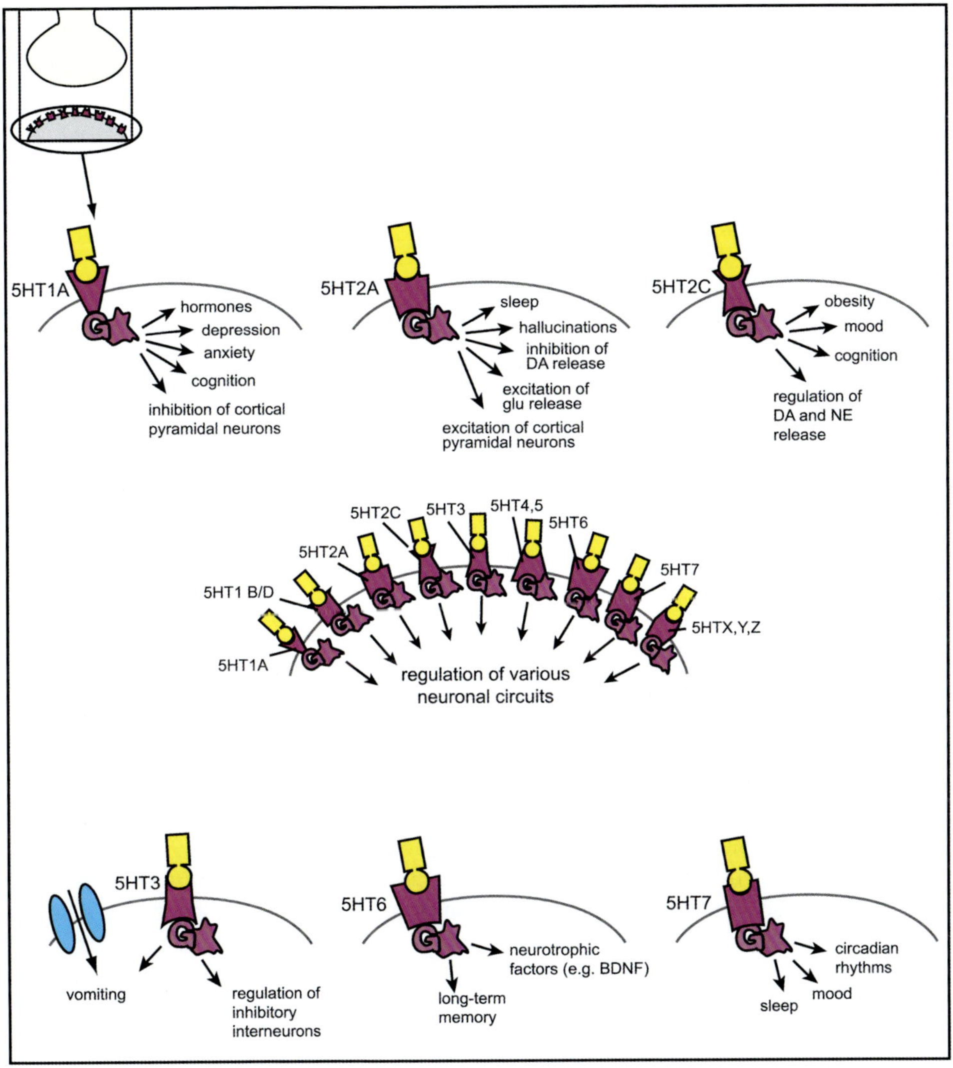

FIGURE 1.18. This figure illustrates various postsynaptic 5HT receptors. Signal transduction and downstream events caused by 5HT binding at these receptors regulate the various neuronal circuits shown and are hypothetically linked to the different functions listed.

Serotonin Pathways

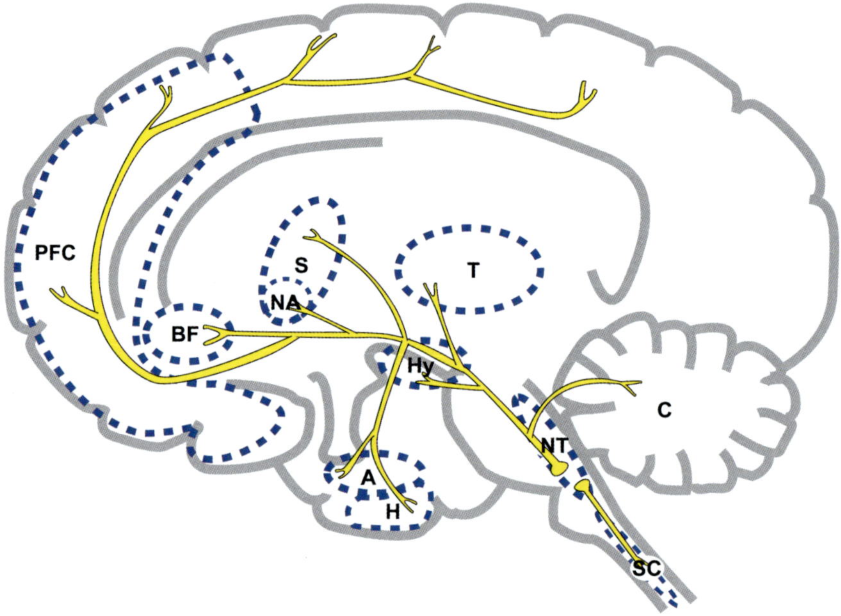

PFC: prefrontal cortex. S: striatum. BF: basal forebrain. NA: nucleus accumbens.T: thalamus. H: hippocampus. Hy: hypothalamus. NT: brain neurotransmitter center. C: cerebellum. SC: spinal cord. A: amygdala.

FIGURE 1.19. These are the major serotonergic projections. Ascending projections originate from raphe nucleus of brainstem to cerebellum, thalamus, hypothalamus, basal forebrain, prefrontal cortex, striatum, nucleus accumbens, amygdala and hippocampus. Mood, appetite, suicidal ideation, and sleep are regulated and affected by 5HT. Descending projections affect pain pathways. Later in this chapter, these circuits will be discussed individually and linked to symptoms of major depressive disorder.

Synthesis and Metabolism of Norepinephrine

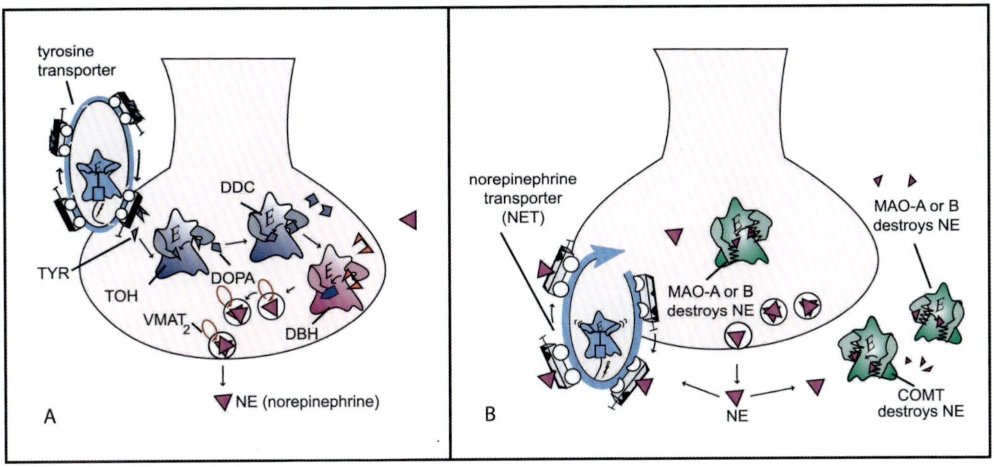

FIGURE 1.20. Norepinephrine (NE) is synthesized from the amino acid tyrosine (TYR), which is transported into the norepinephrine neuron by the tyrosine transporter (A), a transporter that is distinct from the norepinephrine transporter (NET or norepinephrine reuptake pump) shown in B. After tyrosine is pumped into the NE neuron, it is hydroxylated to DOPA by the rate-limiting enzyme for NE synthesis, namely, tyrosine hydroxylase (TOH) (A). DOPA is then decarboxylated to DA by the enzyme DOPA decarboxylase (DDC) (A). In the DA neuron, synthesis stops here. However, in the NE neuron, DA is hydroxylated to NE by the enzyme dopamine beta hydroxylase (DBH) (A), which is actually located at synaptic vesicles. Once synthesized, NE is stored in synaptic vesicles that transport NE inside the vesicles via the vesicular monoamine transporter 2 (VMAT2), also known as the synaptic vesicle pump for monoamines (B).

NE released into the synapse during neurotransmission is either transported back into the NE neuron or metabolized and destroyed extraneuronally by either MAO-A, MAO-B (monoamine oxidase) or COMT (catechol-O-methyl transferase) (B). If NE inside the neuron is not quickly transported into synaptic vesicles (A), it will be destroyed by MAO-A or MAO-B inside the neuron (B).

Norepinephrine Receptors: Part 1

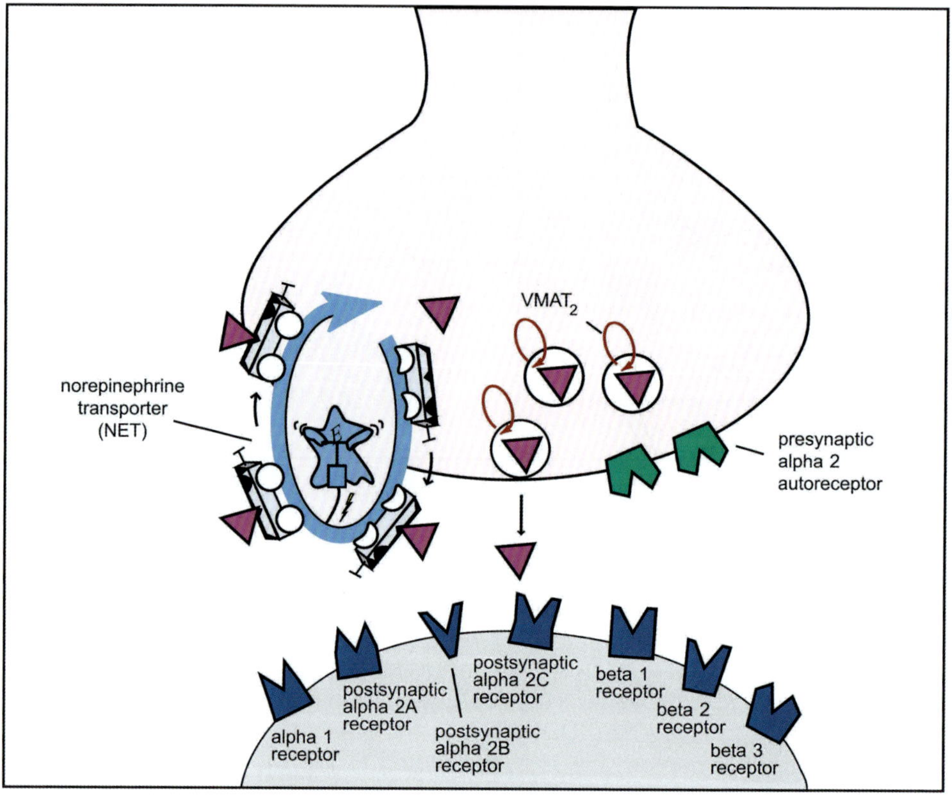

FIGURE 1.21. The norepinephrine transporter (NET) is a presynaptic receptor that clears excess norepinephrine out of the synapse. The synaptic vesicle pump (VMAT2 or vesicular monoamine transporter 2) takes norepinephrine up into synaptic vesicles and stores it for future use. Alpha 2 adrenergic autoreceptors regulate presynaptic norepinephrine release. Postsynaptic norepinephrine receptors also include various subtypes of alpha 2 adrenergic receptors, but also alpha 1 adrenergic receptors and various subtypes of beta adrenergic receptors.

Norepinephrine Receptors: Part 2

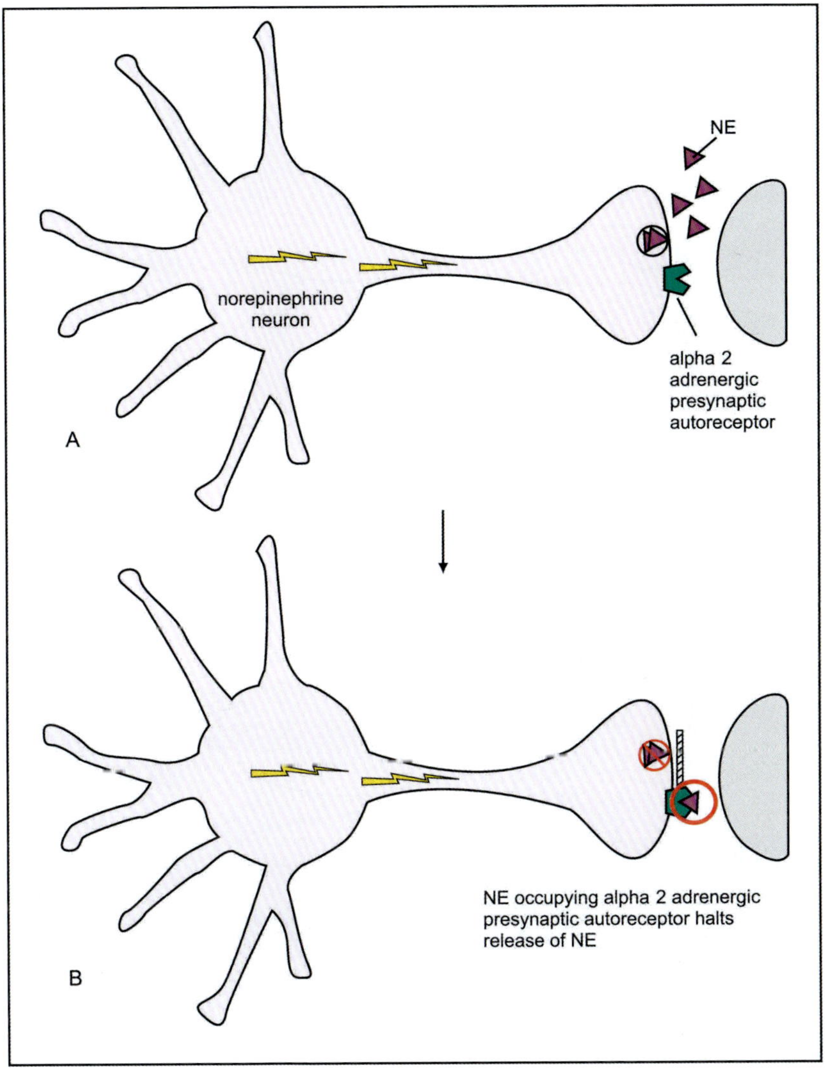

FIGURE 1.22. Presynaptic alpha 2 norepinephrine receptors on the NE neuron's axon terminals work similarly to the 5HT1B/D receptors, acting as "gatekeepers" for their neurotransmitter. When they are not bound by norepinephrine, the gate is open and neurotransmission is allowed to flow (A). When receptors are occupied by the neurotransmitter, further release is prevented (B) (see Fig. 1.16).

Norepinephrine Receptors: Part 3

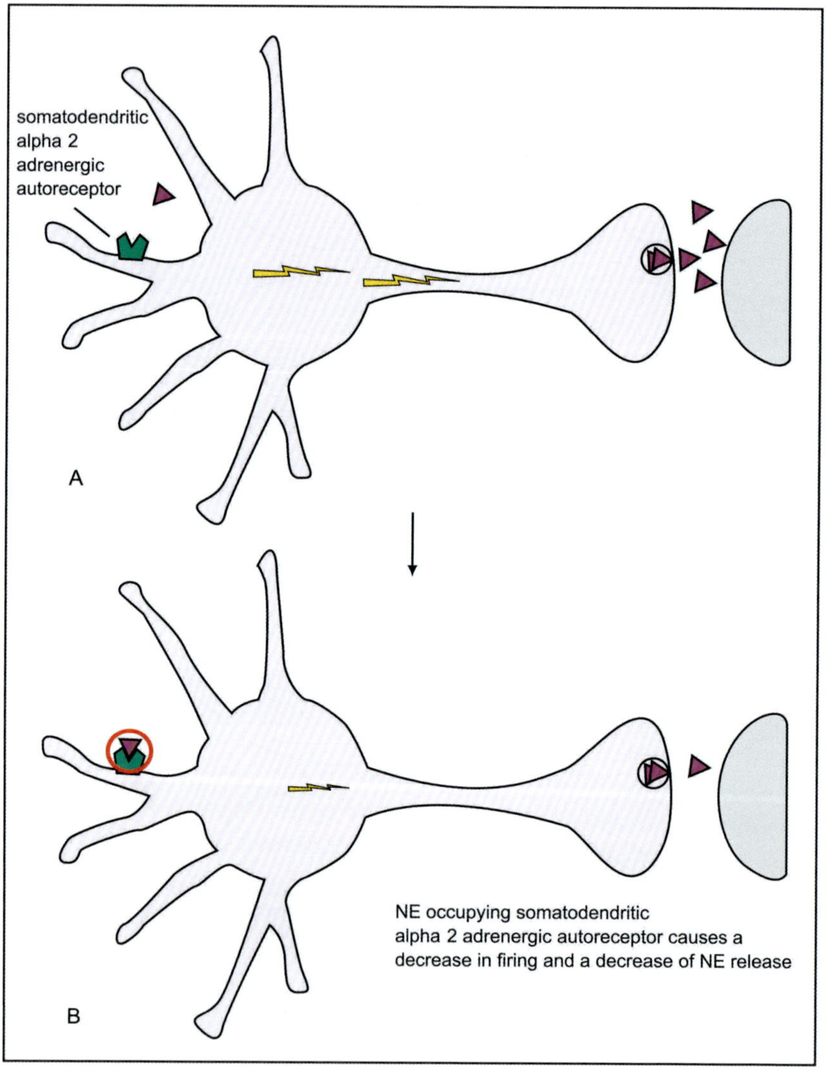

FIGURE 1.23. Presynaptic alpha 2 adrenergic somatodendritic autoreceptors work similarly to somatodendritic 5HT1A receptors, shutting down impulse flow when they are bound by their neurotransmitter (see Fig. 1.17).

Norepinephrine Pathways

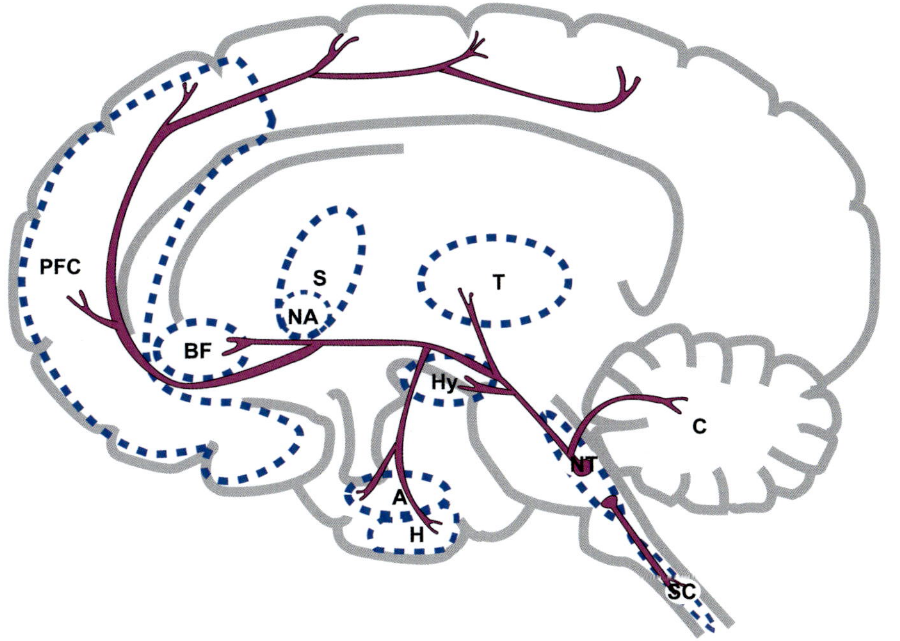

PFC: prefrontal cortex. BF: basal forebrain. NA: nucleus accumbens. T: thalamus. Hy: hypothalamus. A: amygdala. H: hippocampus. C: cerebellum. SC: spinal cord. NT: brain neurotransmitter center. S: striatum

FIGURE 1.24. These are the major norepinephrine pathways. Ascending projections originate from locus coeruleus of brainstem to cerebellum, thalamus, hypothalamus, basal forebrain, prefrontal cortex, amygdala and hippocampus. Mood, arousal and cognition are regulated and affected by NE. Descending projections from the spinal cord affect pain pathways. Later in this chapter, these circuits will be discussed individually and linked to symptoms of major depressive disorder.

Norepinephrine and Serotonin Interactions—NE Regulation of 5HT: Part 1

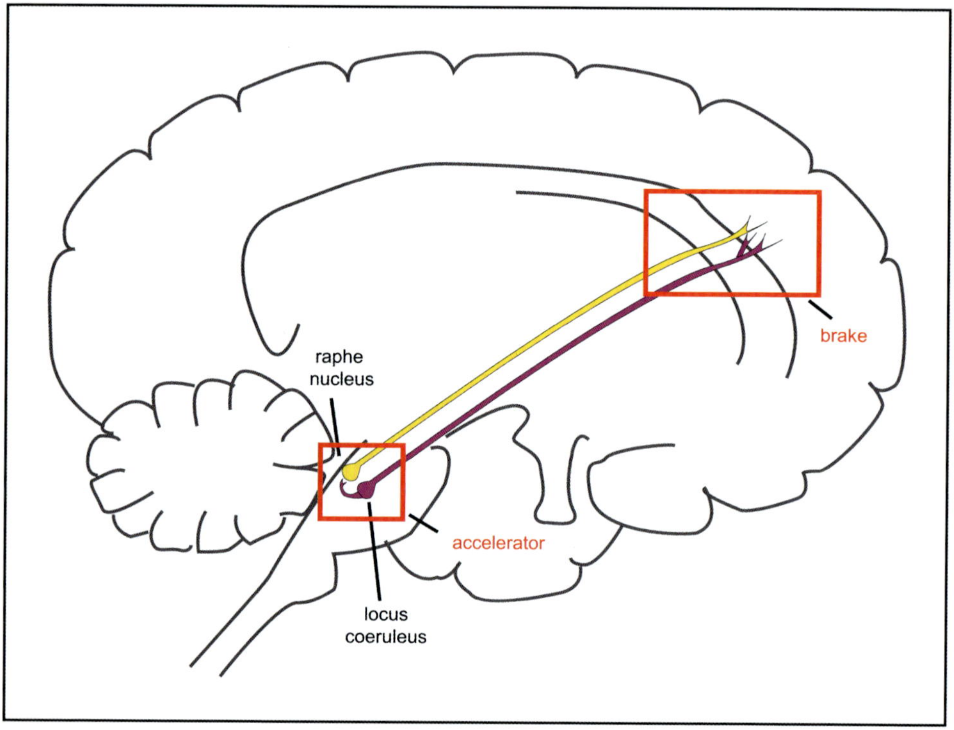

FIGURE 1.25. Norepinephrine can boost 5HT release via an excitatory input from the locus coeruleus projecting to the raphe and acting at alpha 1 receptors on serotonergic cell bodies and dendrites in the raphe. Norepinephrine can also reduce 5HT release via an inhibitory input from NE nerve terminals acting at 5HT nerve terminals on alpha 2 receptors on serotonin axon terminals (5HT brake).

Norepinephrine and Serotonin Interactions—NE Regulation of 5HT: Part 2

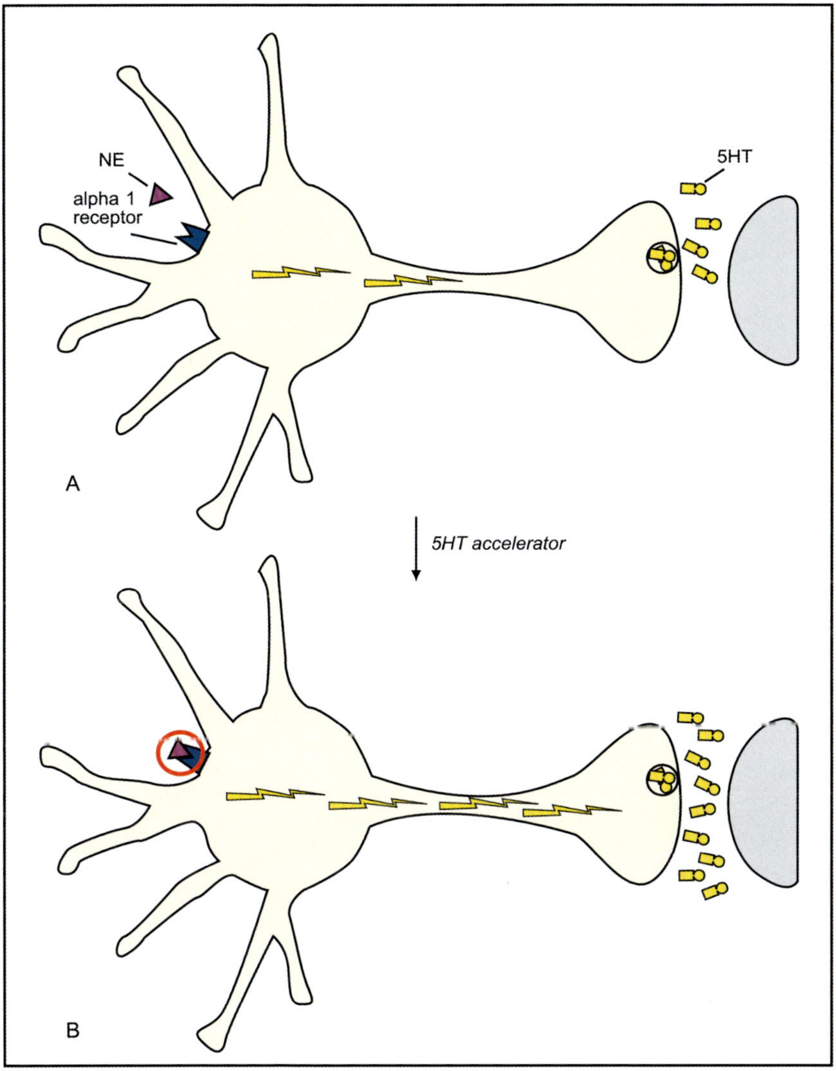

FIGURE 1.26. A close-up of the 5HT accelerator is shown here, where NE occupies alpha 1 receptors on somatodendritic areas of serotonin cell bodies (A). This causes excitation of the 5HT neuron, with increased neuronal impulse flow and increased release of 5HT from its axon terminals (B).

Norepinephrine and Serotonin Interactions—NE Regulation of 5HT: Part 3

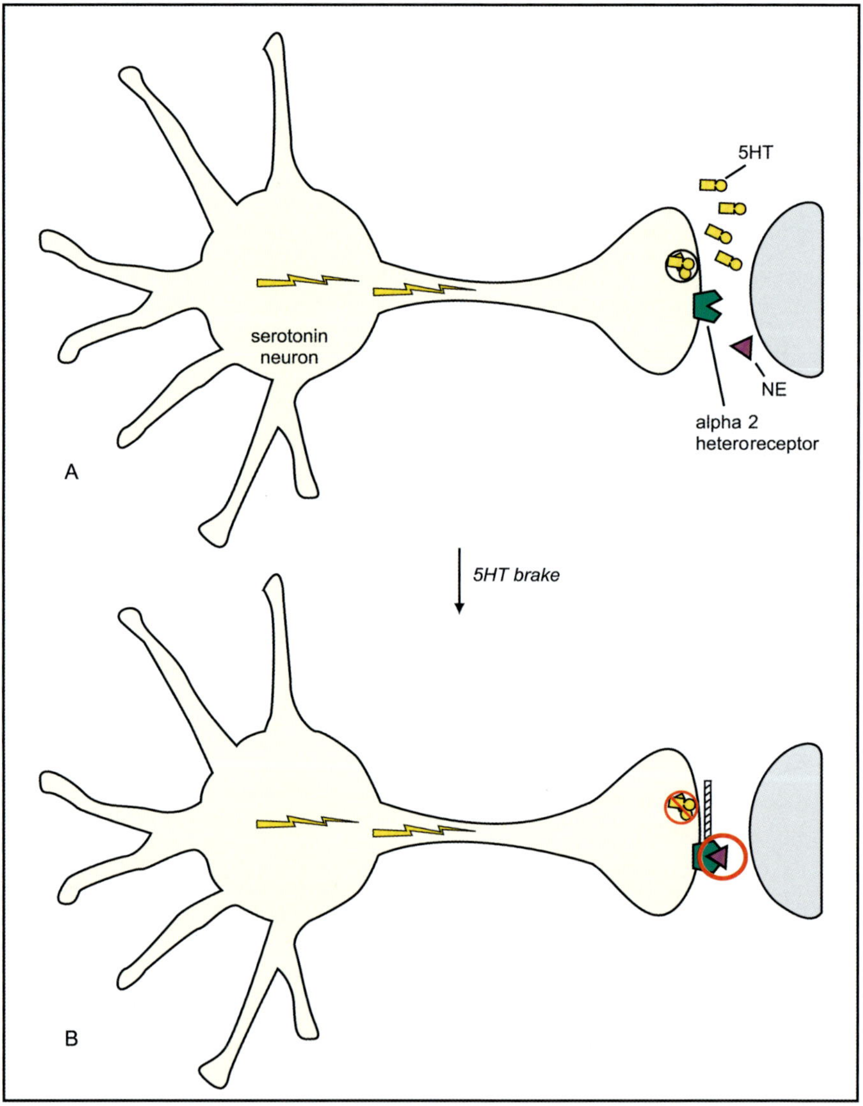

FIGURE 1.27. A close-up of the 5HT brake is shown, where NE occupies alpha 2 heteroreceptors for NE on 5HT axon terminals (A). This causes inhibition of 5HT release from the 5HT neuron (B).

Synthesis and Metabolism of Dopamine

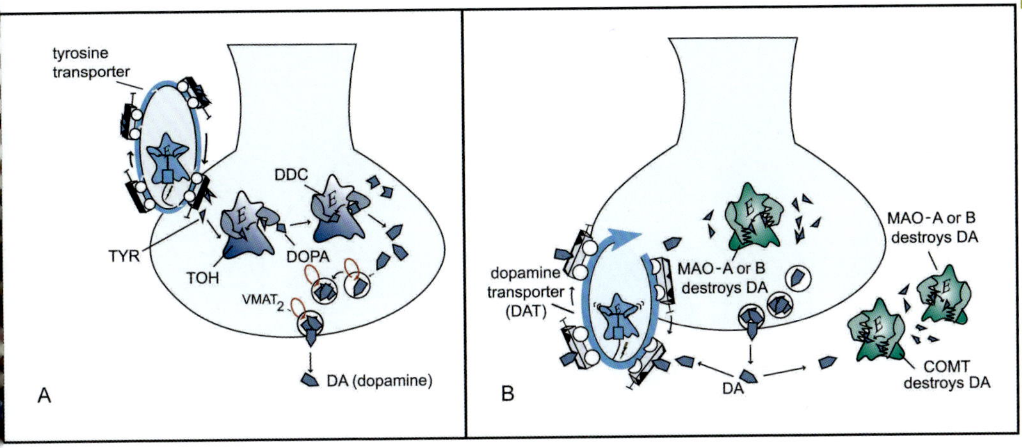

FIGURE 1.28. Dopamine (DA) is synthesized from the amino acid tyrosine (TYR), which is transported into the DA neuron by the tyrosine transporter (A), a transporter that is distinct from the DA transporter shown in B. After tyrosine is pumped into the DA neuron, it is hydroxylated to DOPA by the rate-limiting enzyme for DA synthesis; namely, tyrosine hydroxylase (TOH) (A). DOPA is then decarboxylated to DA by the enzyme DOPA decarboxylase (DDC) (A). DA synthesized in the presynaptic neuron is then transported into synaptic vesicles via the synaptic vesicle pump VMAT2 (vesicular monoamine transporter 2) (A). There it is stored until released during neurotransmission (B).

DA released into the synapse during neurotransmission is either transported back into the DA neuron or metabolized and destroyed by either monoamine oxidase (MAO)-A or MAO-B, or COMT (catechol-O-methyl transferase) (B). If DA inside the neuron is not quickly transported into synaptic vesicles (A), it will be destroyed by MAO-A or MAO-B inside the neuron (B).

Dopamine Receptors: Part 1

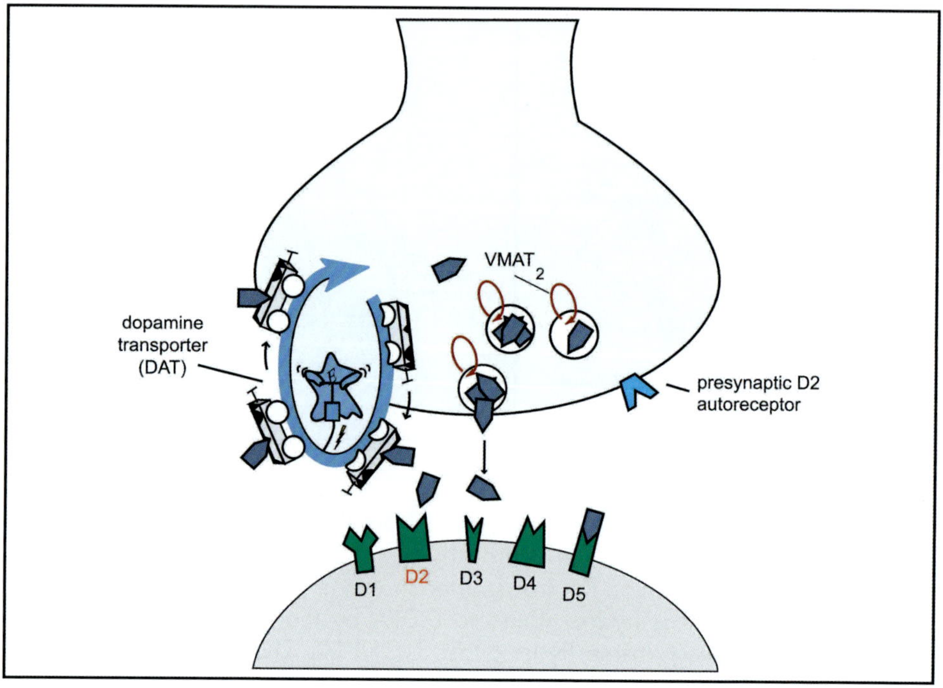

FIGURE 1.29. DA receptors that regulate dopaminergic neurotransmission are depicted. The dopamine transporter (DAT) is presynaptic and removes excess DA from the synapse. VMAT2 (vesicular monoamine transporter 2) transports DA into synaptic vesicles for future transmission. A presynaptic D2 autoreceptor regulates DA release. Postsynaptic DA receptors include D1, D2, D3, D4 and D5. D2 is most studied due to its role as a primary binding site for antipsychotic agents and dopamine agonists.

Dopamine Receptors: Part 2

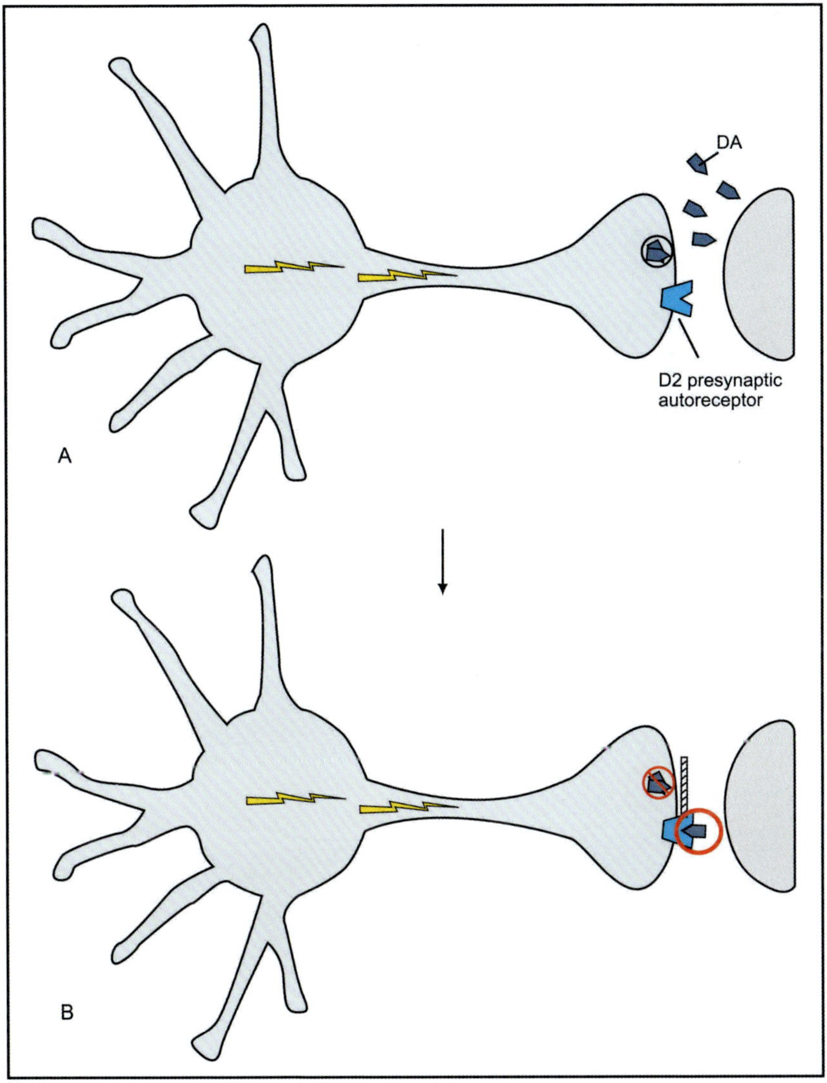

FIGURE 1.30. Presynaptic dopamine 2 receptors on the DA neuron's axon terminals act as "gatekeepers" for their neurotransmitter. When they are not bound by DA, the gate is open and neurotransmission is allowed to flow (A). When receptors are occupied by DA, further release is prevented (B).

Dopamine Receptors: Part 3

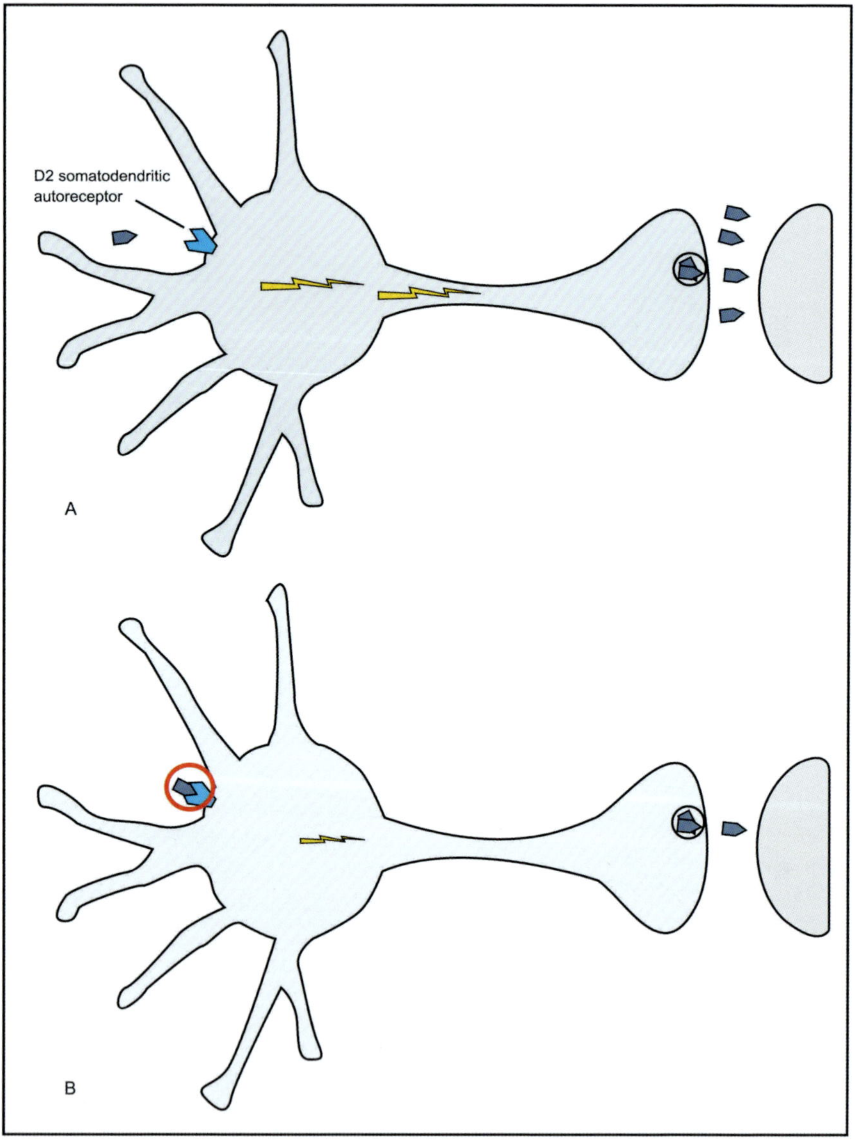

FIGURE 1.31. Presynaptic dopamine 2 somatodendritic autoreceptors (A) work by shutting down impulse flow when they are bound by their neurotransmitter (DA) (B).

Serotonin – Dopamine Interactions:
5HT2A and 5HT1A Receptors Have Opposite Actions on DA Release

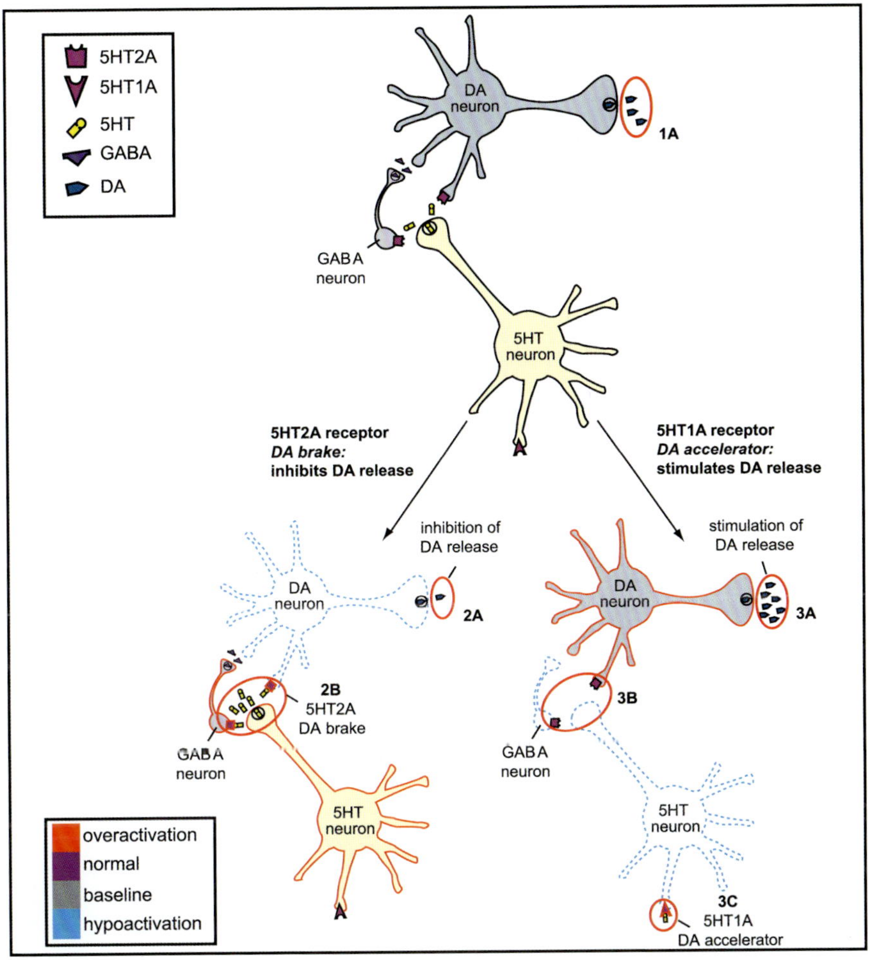

FIGURE 1.32. 5HT1A and 5HT2A receptors both affect DA release. 5HT2A receptors act as a brake for DA, inhibiting release (compare 2A to 1A) when 5HT binds to 5HT2A receptors on postsynaptic DA neurons (2B). This same effect occurs when 5HT binds to 5HT2A receptors on GABA interneurons (2B), releasing GABA and inhibiting DA (2A). However, when 5HT binds to 5HT1A receptors (3C), serotonin release is inhibited (3B) (see Fig. 1.17). This removes the inhibitory effect of 5HT on DA neurons at postysynaptic 5HT2A receptors. Thus, DA release is disinhibited, resulting in an increase of DA (3A).

Serotonin – Dopamine – Norepinephrine Interactions: 5HT2C Receptors Reduce Release of DA and NE in Prefrontal Cortex

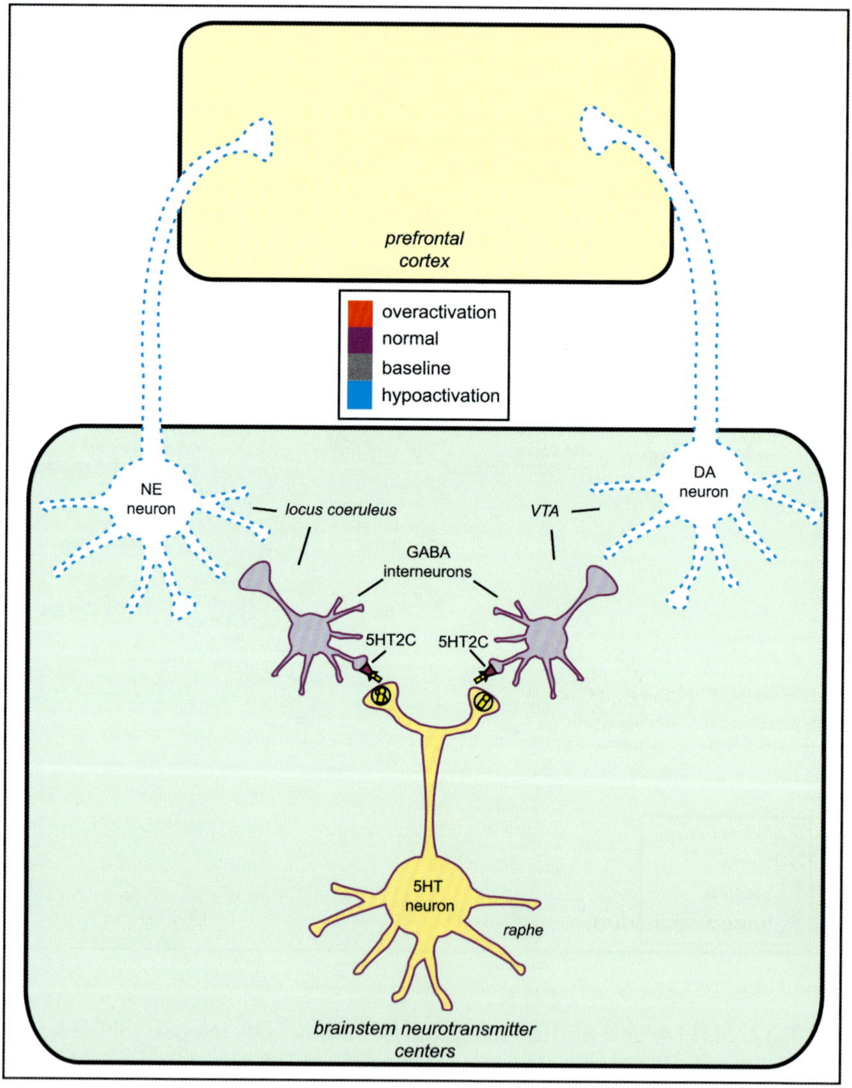

FIGURE 1.33. 5HT2C receptors inhibit both DA and NE release. This occurs when 5HT binds to 5HT2C receptors on GABA interneurons in the brainstem and excites them, causing release of the inhibitory neurotransmitter GABA onto both NE neurons (on the left) and DA neurons (on the right).

Dopamine Pathways

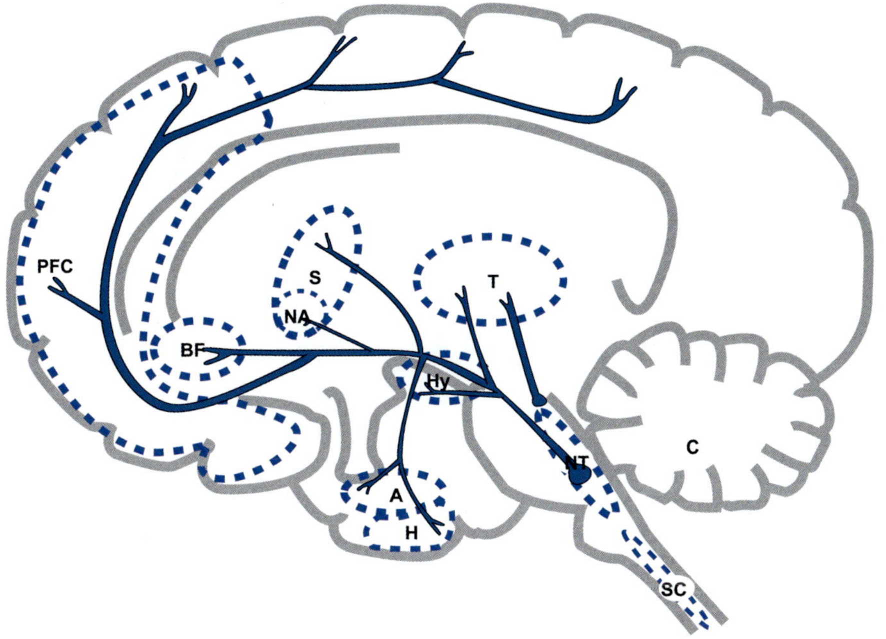

PFC: prefrontal cortex. S: striatum. BF: basal forebrain. NA: nucleus accumbens. Hy: hypothalamus. T: thalamus. H: hippocampus. A: amygdala. C: cerebellum. SC: spinal cord. NT: brain neurotransmitter center.

FIGURE 1.34. Dopamine projections ascend to several brain regions from the brainstem. Dopaminergic neurotransmission is associated with cognition, psychosis, pleasure and reward, movement and other functions. Later in this chapter, these circuits will be discussed individually and linked to symptoms of major depressive disorder.

Circuits and Symptoms in Depression:
Part 1, Affect-Meter and Monoamines

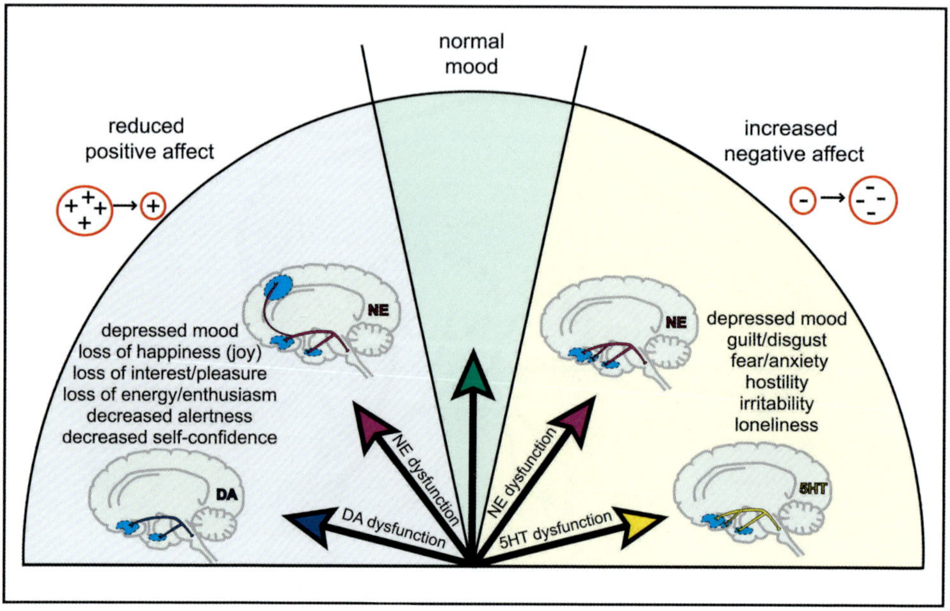

FIGURE 1.35. Depression involves a variety of mood-related symptoms that represent either decreased positive affect (on the left) or increased negative affect (on the right). When positive affect is reduced, symptoms on the left of the affect-meter may be observed, with dopaminergic and noradrenergic dysfunction hypothetically playing a role. When negative affect is increased, symptoms on the right half of the affect-meter may be observed, with theoretical serotonergic and noradrenergic dysfunction.

Circuits and Symptoms in Depression:

Part 2, Matching Symptoms to Circuits

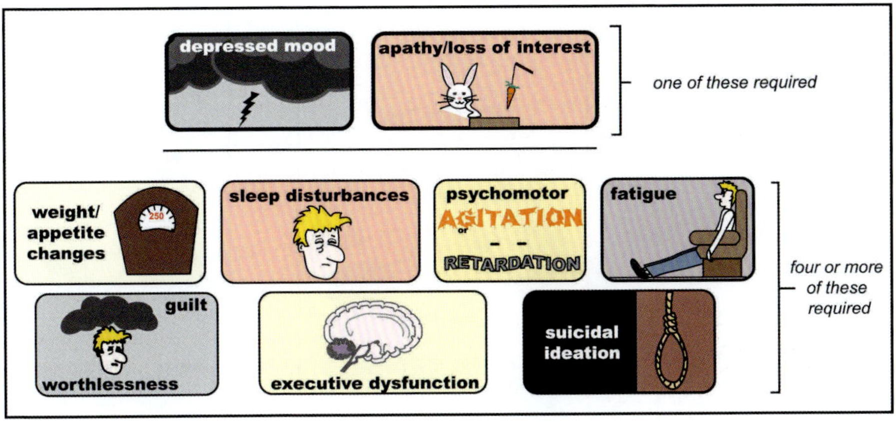

FIGURE 1.36. The symptoms required for a DSM-IV (Diagnostic and Statistical Manual, version IV) diagnosis for major depressive disorder (MDD).

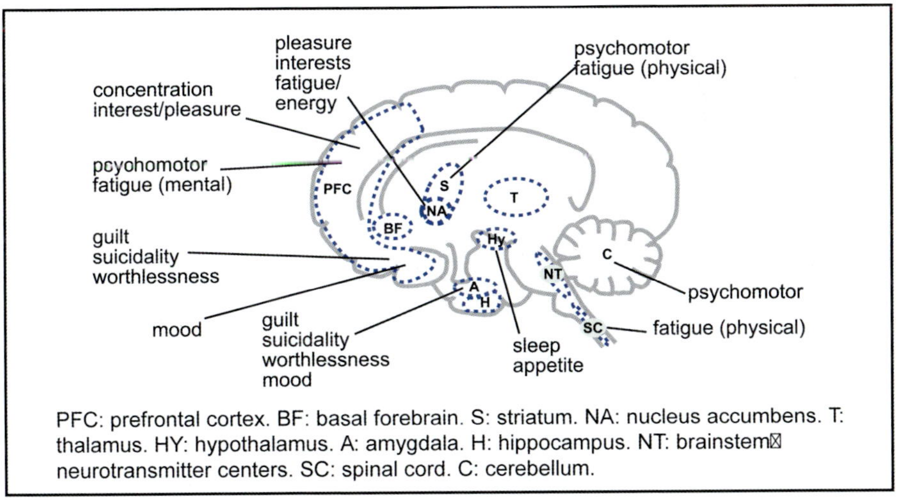

FIGURE 1.37. Malfunctioning of brain regions shown above may hypothetically be altered due to aberrant neuronal activity and information processing, leading to the different presenting symptoms of depression. Circuits may manifest hypo- or hyperactivity. For simplicity, future pages indicate hypoactivity in blue and hyperactivity in red.

Circuits and Symptoms in Depression: Part 3

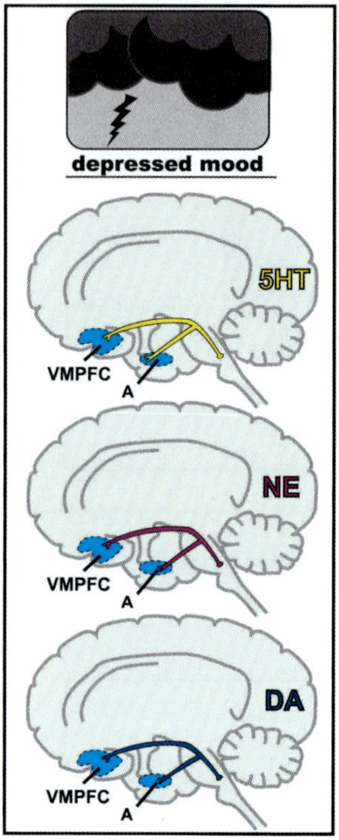

FIGURE 1.38. Inefficient or dysfunctional serotonin (5HT), norepinephrine (NE), and/or dopamine (DA) projections to the amygdala (A) and ventromedial prefrontal cortex (VMPFC) are hypothetically linked to depressed mood.

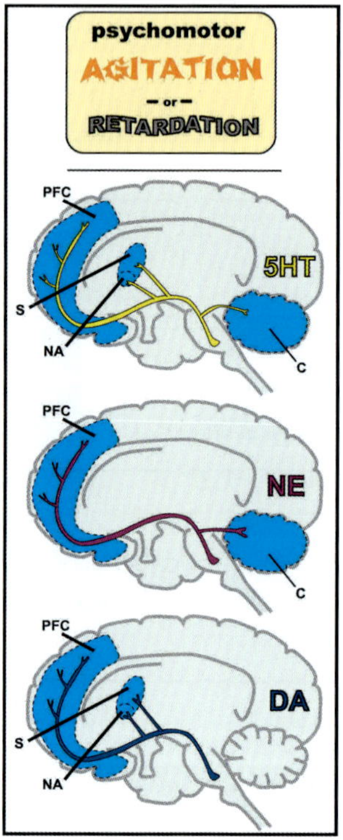

FIGURE 1.39. Inefficient information processing in the cerebellum (C) (5HT and NE projections), striatum (S) and nucleus accumbens (NA) (5HT and DA projections), and the PFC (projections of all three monoamines) is hypothetically linked to psychomotor agitation or retardation.

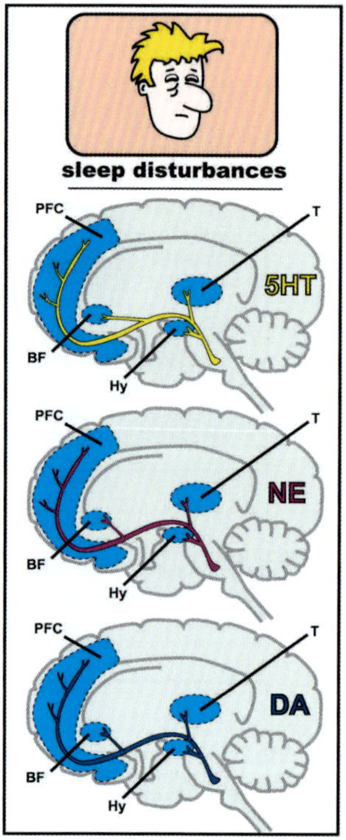

FIGURE 1.40. All three monoamines project from brainstem nuclei to the hypothalamus (Hy), thalamus (T), basal forebrain (BF), and PFC. Hypoactivation of these four areas is hypothetically linked to sleep disturbances.

Circuits and Symptoms in Depression: Part 4

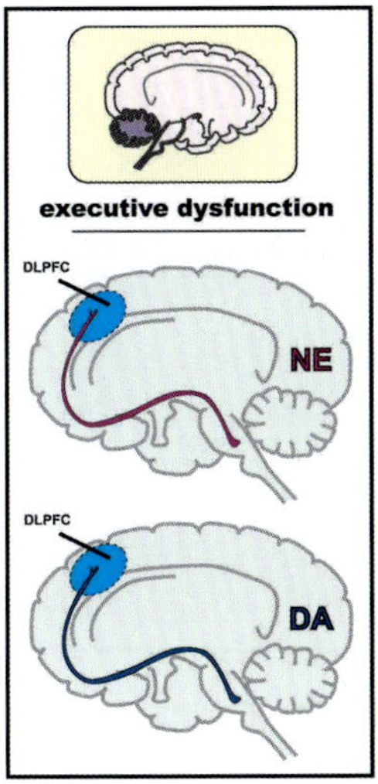

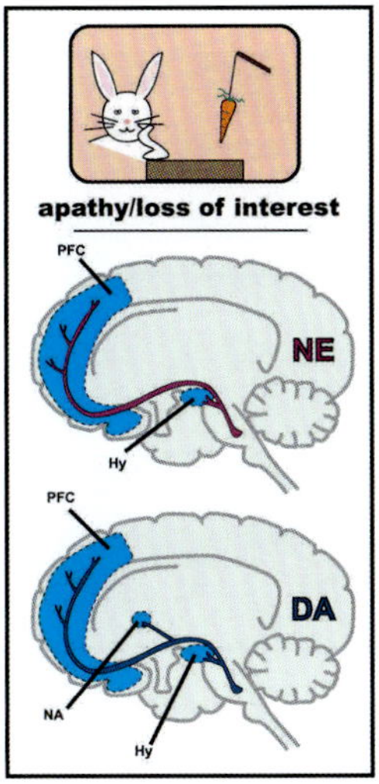

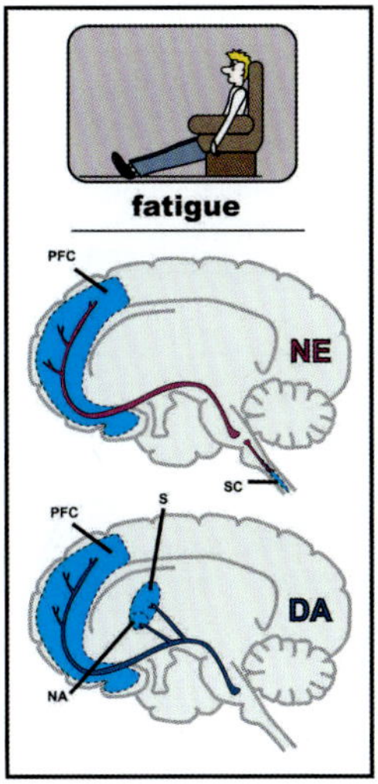

FIGURE 1.41. Inefficient information processing, particularly from the NE and DA projections to the dorsolateral prefrontal cortex (DLPFC) are hypothetically linked to symptoms involving executive dysfunction, including emotional regulation, self-monitoring, goal-setting, priority planning, and organization.

FIGURE 1.42. Apathy, although superficially similar to depressed mood, is actually a distinct symptom of depression, associated with lack of pleasure including decreased libido, linked to loss of interest and motivation and often experienced by geriatric patients. Apathy is also hypothetically regulated by different brain circuits than depressed mood. These are the NE projections to the PFC and Hy and the DA projections to the PFC, Hy, and NA.

FIGURE 1.43. Mental fatigue is linked to inefficient information processing of NE and DA in the PFC. Physical fatigue is linked to deficient NE functioning in the descending spinal cord (SC) and deficient DA functioning in the striatum (S), NA and Hy.

Circuits and Symptoms in Depression: Part 5

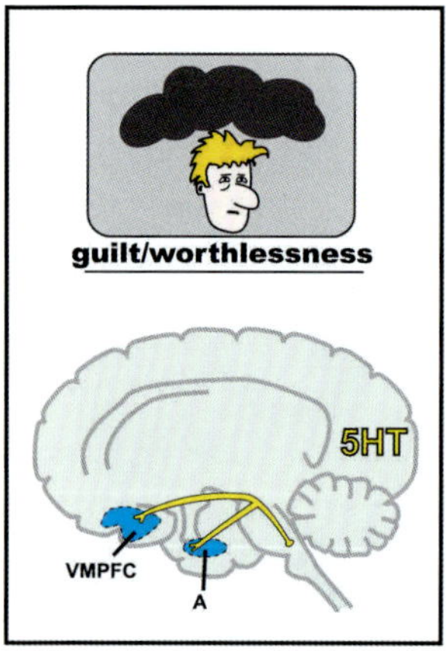

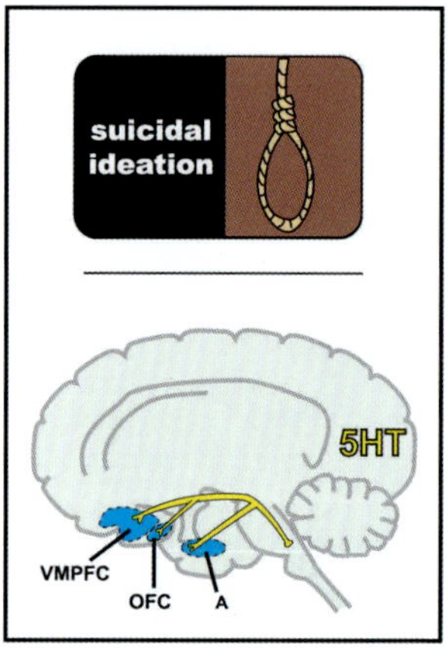

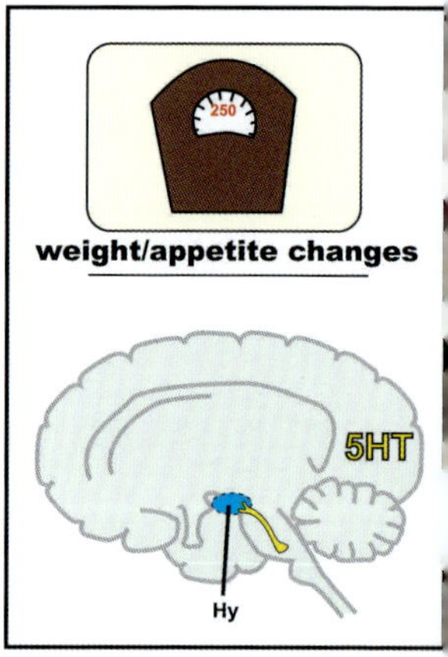

FIGURE 1.44. Feelings of guilt and worthlessness are hypothetically regulated by the amygdala and VMPFC, which are known as "emotional" brain regions. Inefficient or dysfunctional 5HT projections to these areas could theoretically cause these symptoms.

FIGURE 1.45. Suicidal ideation, is hypothetically regulated by 5HT control of "emotional" brain regions including the amygdala, VMPFC, and orbital frontal cortex (OFC).

FIGURE 1.46. Weight and appetite are hypothetically regulated largely by 5HT projections to the Hy.

Circuits and Symptoms in Depression:
Part 6, Neuroimaging of Brain Activation in Depression

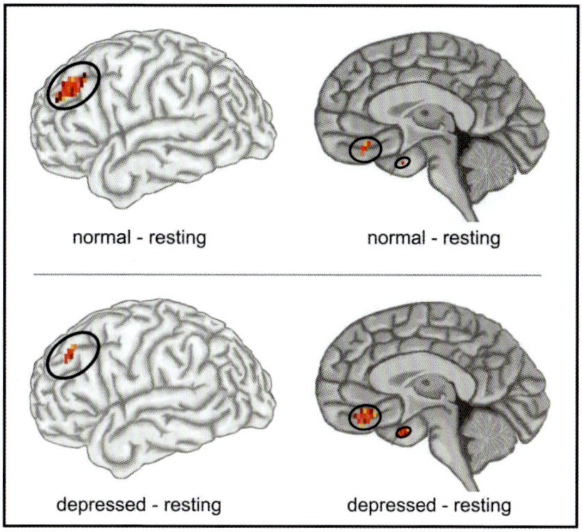

FIGURE 1.47. Neuroimaging studies indicate that activity in the dorsolateral prefrontal cortex (DLPFC) is decreased in depressed patients, whereas amygdala and ventromedial prefrontal cortex (VMPFC) functioning are increased at rest.

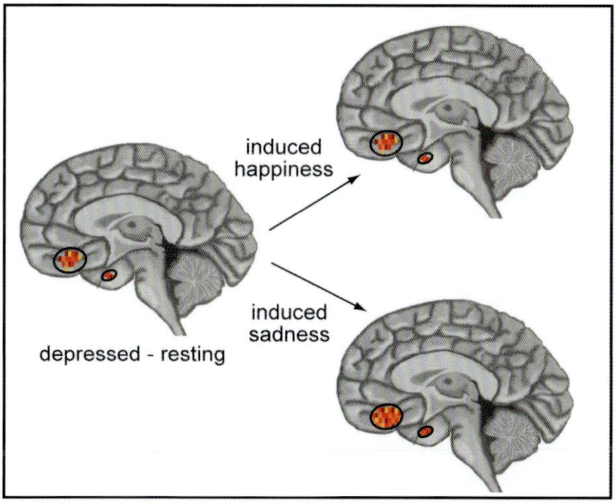

FIGURE 1.48. Depressed patients show over-activation of VMPFC and amygdala in response to induced sadness and under-activation in response to induced happiness.

From Genes to Circuits to Symptoms

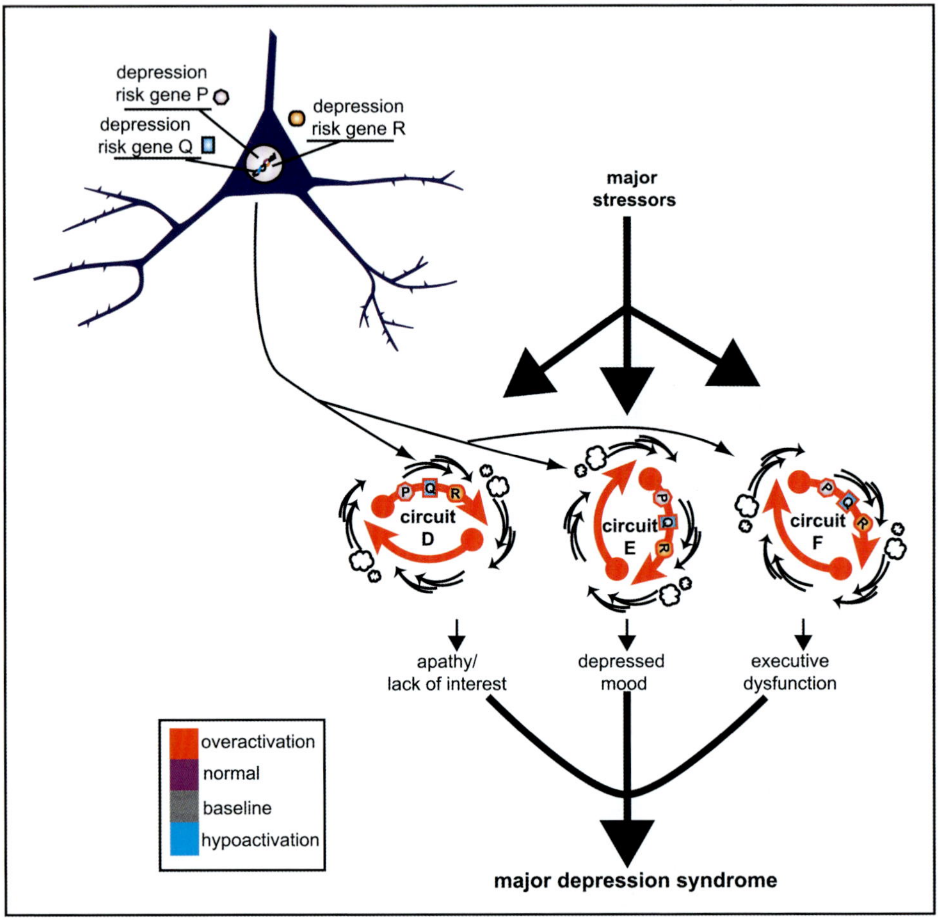

FIGURE 1.49. Major depressive disorder (MDD) may not be inherited per se, but risk for MDD may be inherited as a series of risk genes (indicated here as P, Q and R). Whether this risk manifests itself as overt MDD may depend upon exposure of genetically vulnerable circuits to stress. In the presence of major stressors, circuits rendered vulnerable by risk genes to developing inefficient information processing under stress may break down, and if sufficient symptoms prevail, MDD may result.

Stahl's Illustrated | Chapter 2

Selective Serotonin Reuptake Inhibitors (SSRIs) and Serotonin Norepinephrine Reuptake Inhibitors (SNRIs)

This chapter reviews some of the most commonly used first-line antidepressant drug options, the selective serotonin reuptake inhibitors (SSRIs) and serotonin norepinephrine reuptake inhibitors (SNRIs). For patients who do not completely remit on an SSRI or SNRI, oftentimes augmentation and/or combinations are introduced or the patient is switched to a second-line treatment. This concept is developed in further detail in later chapters. Here, each of the six drugs in the SSRI class and each of the four drugs in the SNRI class is reviewed.

Symbols Used in this Chapter			
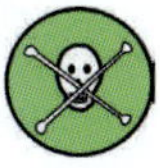	Life-threatening or Dangerous Side Effects	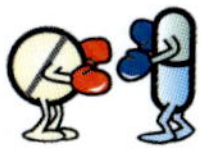	Drug Interactions
	Tips and Pearls		Cardiac Impairment
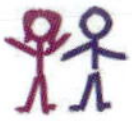	Children and Adolescents	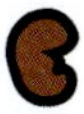	Renal Impairment
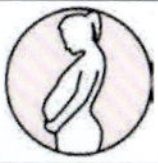	Pregnancy	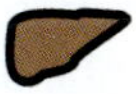	Hepatic Impairment

SSRIs and SNRIs as First-Line Treatments

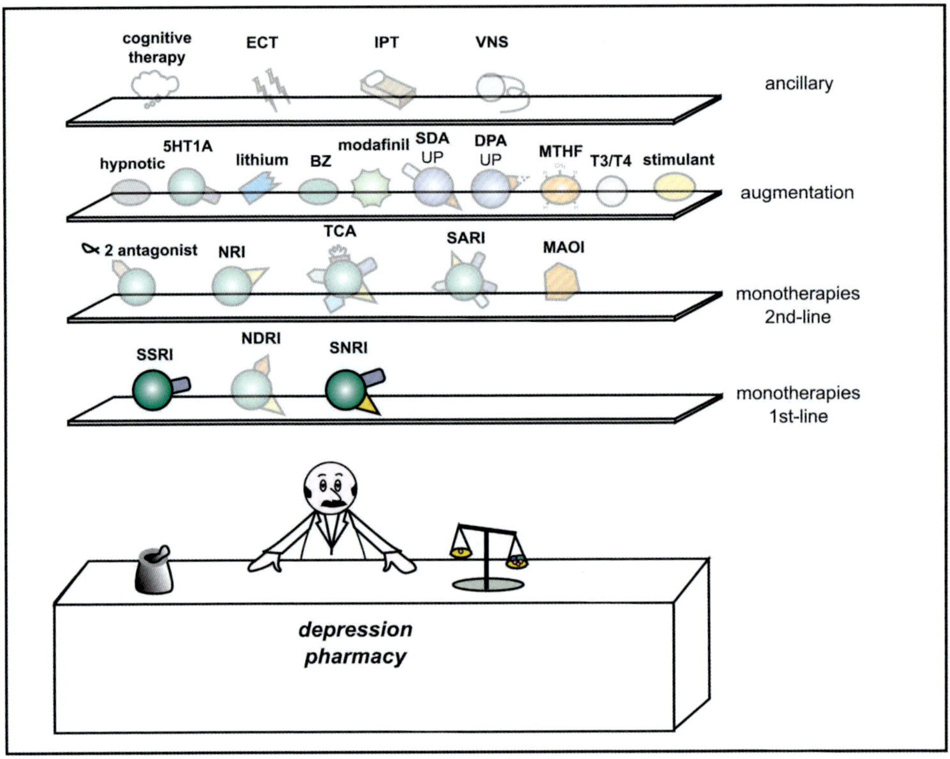

FIGURE 2.1. The depression pharmacy is full of various treatment options used in the management of depression. Here, only SSRIs and SNRIs are highlighted on the shelf to indicate that these treatments are first-line monotherapies. This figure will be utilized throughout the book to indicate where on the pharmacy shelves the various pharmacotherapies under discussion fall in the sequence of selecting treatments for depression.

SSRI: selective serotonin reuptake inhibitors. NDRI: norepinephrine dopamine reuptake inhibitors. SNRI: serotonin norepinephrine reuptake inhibitors. SDA: serotonin dopamine antagonists. α 2 antagonist: alpha 2 antagonists. NRI: selective norepinephrine reuptake inhibitors. TCA: tricyclic antidepressants. SARI: serotonin 2A antagonist/reuptake inhibitors. MAOI: monoamine oxidase inhibitors. 5HT1A: serotonin 1A partial agonists. BZ: benzodiazepines. DPA: dopamine partial agonists. MTHF: L-5-methyl-tetrahydrofolate. T3/T4: thyroid hormone. ECT: electroconvulsive therapy. IPT: interpersonal therapy. VNS: vagus nerve stimulation.

Selective Serotonin Reuptake Inhibitors (SSRIs):
Mechanism of Action (Pharmacological and Molecular)

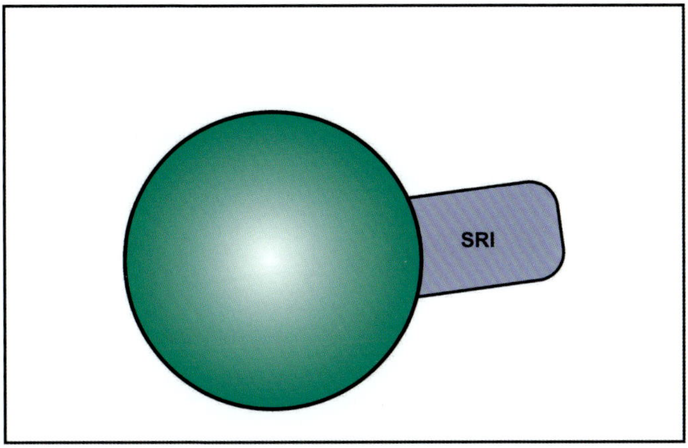

FIGURE 2.2. The core feature of SSRIs is serotonin reuptake inhibition (SRI, indicated above). Six agents are in the SSRI class; each shares the common property of serotonin transporter (SERT) inhibition.

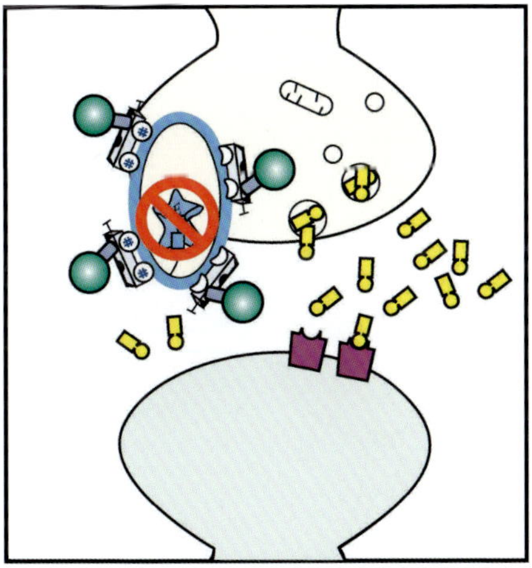

FIGURE 2.3. As depicted above, the SRI property of SSRIs takes place at the SERT, binding to it and preventing 5HT from being taken up, thus leaving more neurotransmitter in the synapse and providing an antidepressant effect. The molecular mechanism of action of SSRIs, including downstream effects on receptors, is illustrated in detail on the following pages.

SSRI Molecular Mechanism of Action:

Parts 1 and 2

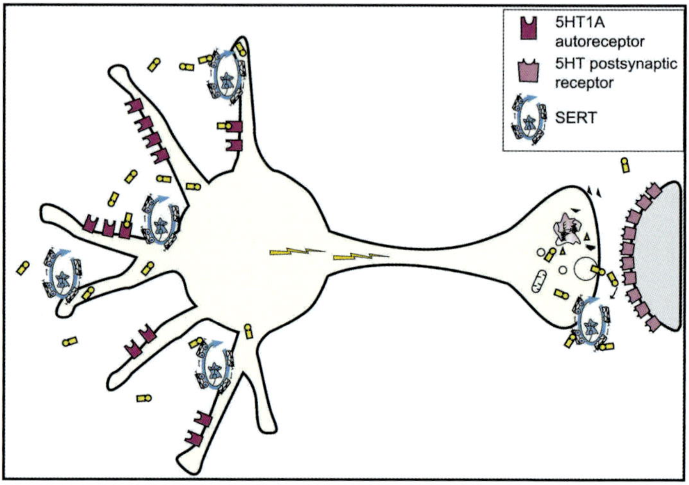

FIGURE 2.4. In the depressed state, there is low 5HT, upregulated receptors and a low number of signals in the neuron to release more 5HT.

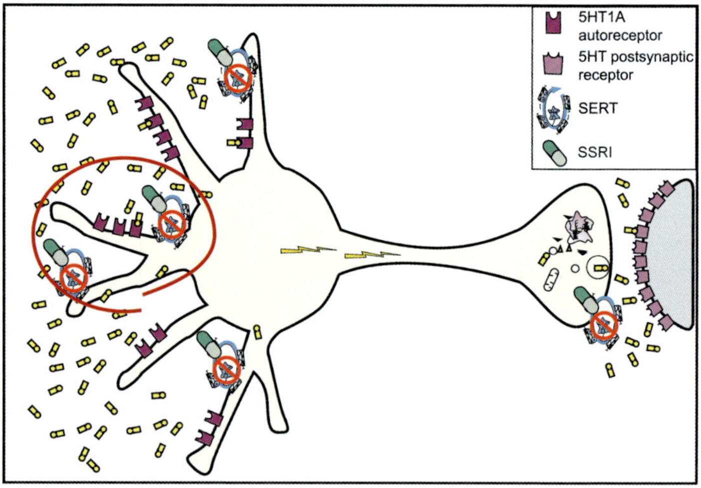

FIGURE 2.5. Antidepressant action: SSRI blocks 5HT reuptake at both the dendrites (red circle on the left) and the axon (on the right).

SSRI Molecular Mechanism of Action:

Parts 3 and 4

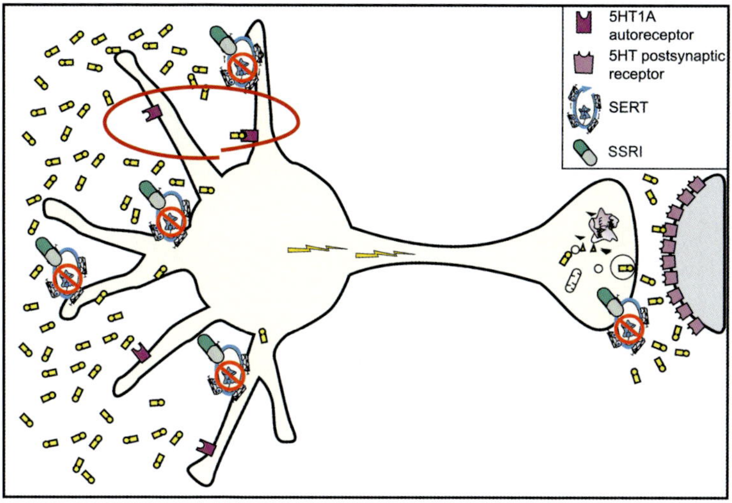

FIGURE 2.6. The increase in 5HT causes the autoreceptors to desensitize/downregulate (red circle on the left) and to increase somatodendritic serotonin release (red circle on the left).

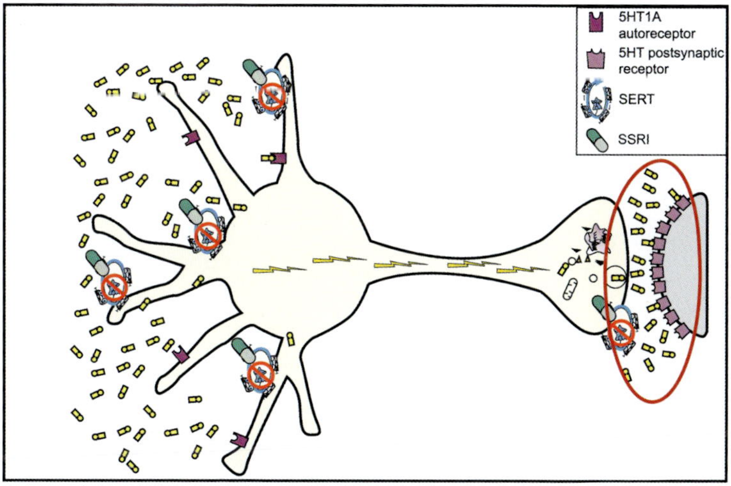

FIGURE 2.7. The downregulation of the autoreceptors causes the neurons to release more 5HT at the axon terminal (red circle on the right).

SSRI Molecular Mechanism of Action:
Part 5

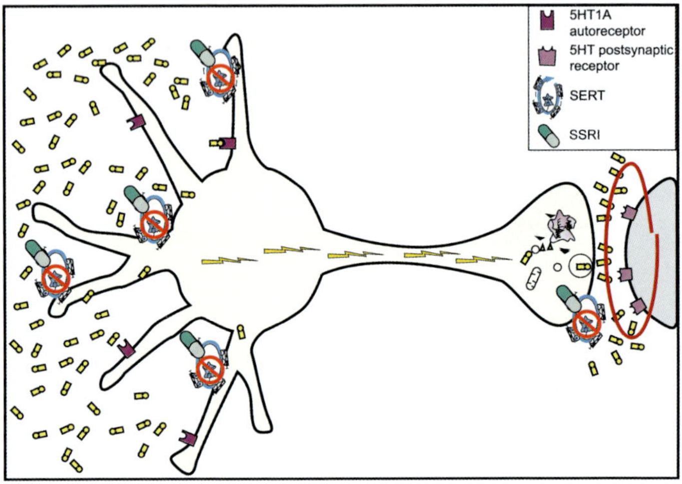

FIGURE 2.8. The increase of 5HT at the axon causes the postsynaptic receptors to desensitize/downregulate, reducing side effects (red circle on the right).

Secondary Pharmacological Actions of SSRIs

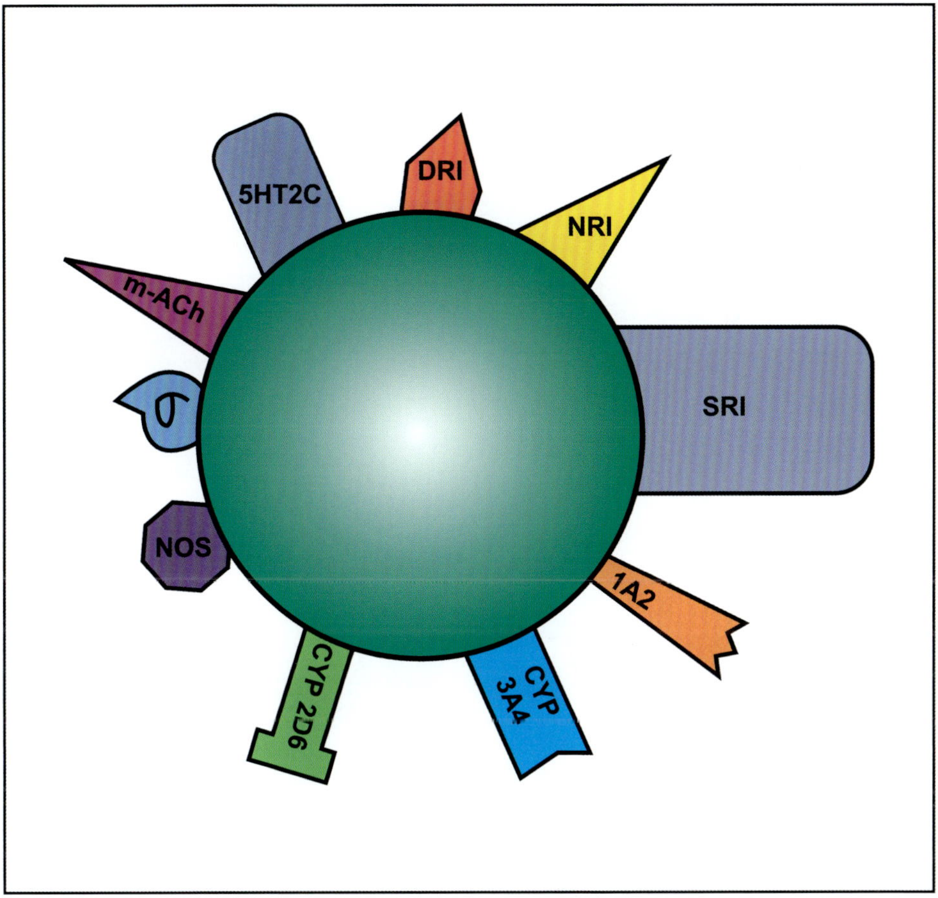

FIGURE 2.9. While SSRIs have in common their high affinity for serotonin reuptake inhibition (SRI), each has different secondary pharmacological actions, which include NRI (norepinephrine reuptake inhibition), DRI (dopamine reuptake inhibition), 5HT2C antagonism, muscarinic/cholinergic antagonism (m-ACh), sigma-1 receptor actions (σ), and inhibition of NOS (nitric oxide synthetase) and of CYP450 2D6, 3A4 and 1A2. Pharmacologic properties of each of the six SSRIs are shown in the following figures.

Fluoxetine

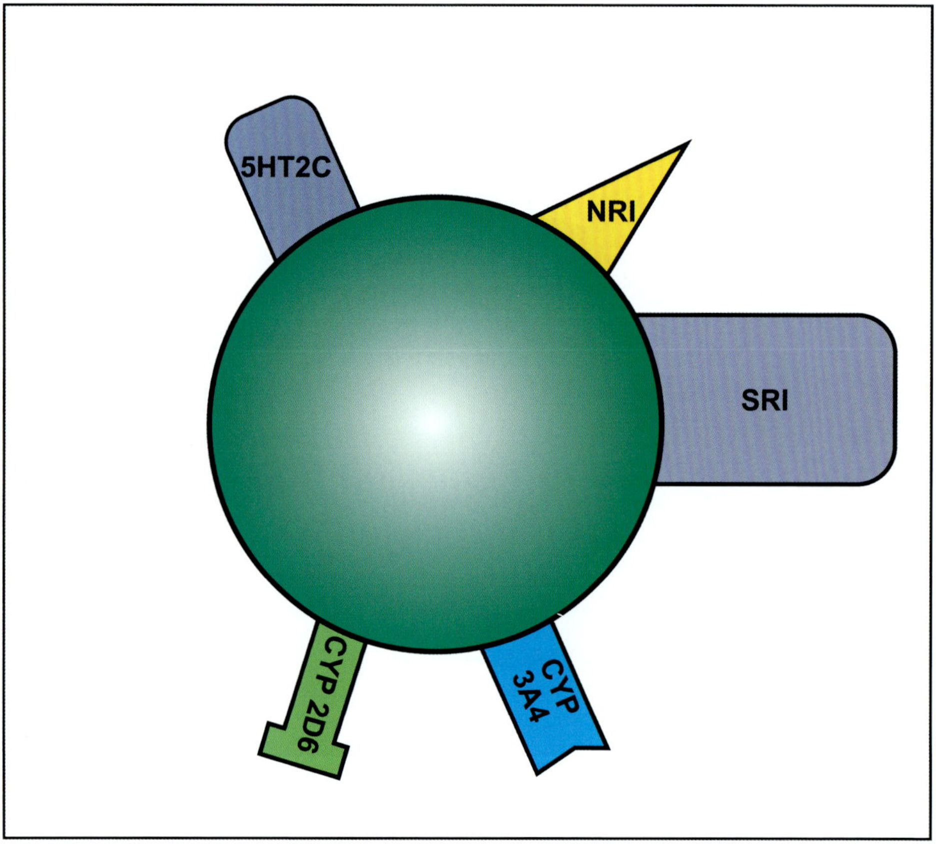

FIGURE 2.10. Fluoxetine has antagonist actions at 5HT2C receptors, which results in NE and DA release. Recall that serotonin normally inhibits DA and NE release at 5HT2C receptors (see Fig. 1.33). Thus, when 5HT2C receptors are blocked, this stops that inhibition; this is also called "disinhibition." Therefore, blocking 5HT2C receptors results in NE and DA disinhibition; 5HT2C antagonists such as fluoxetine are NE and DA disinhibitors, or NDDIs. Fluoxetine also inhibits CYP450 2D6 and 3A4. Fluoxetine has a long half-life, while its active metabolite has an even longer half-life; these factors may reduce the incidence of sudden withdrawal symptoms. Fluoxetine may be useful in conjunction with atypical antipsychotics, including olanzapine, to increase the effectiveness of their antidepressant action for bipolar depression.

Fluoxetine: Tips and Pearls

Dosing

Formulation:
10, 20, 40, 60 mg capsules; 10 mg tablet; 20 mg/5 mL -120 mL bottles liquid. Weekly capsule 90 mg

Dosage Range:
20-80 mg for depression and anxiety. 60-80 mg for bulimia

Approved For:
Major depressive disorder, obsessive compulsive disorder, premenstrual dysphoric disorder, bulimia nervosa, panic disorder, bipolar depression (with olanzapine)

Pearls

May be first-line choice for atypical depression. Actions at 5HT2C receptors may explain activating properties and, in part, efficacy in combination with olanzapine for treatment-resistant depression

Use with caution in children. Watch for induction of mania or suicidal ideation. Children may have slower growth. Approved for use in children with OCD. Only SSRI approved for depression in adolescents

Pregnancy risk category C (some animal studies show adverse effects, no controlled studies in humans)

Side effects I

Weight Gain

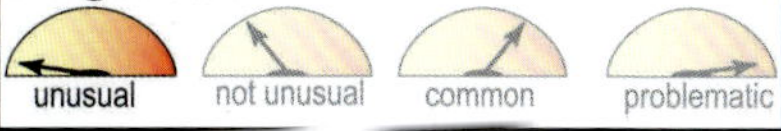

Sedation

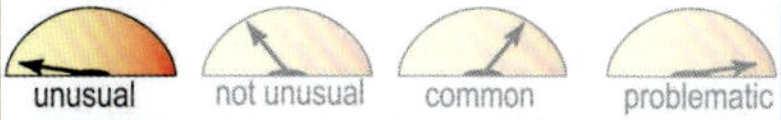

Rare seizures, induction of mania and suicidality

Side effects II

Via CYP450 2D6 and 3A4 inhibition, may increase concentrations of other drugs. Do not use with MAOIs, thioridazine, pimozide

Preliminary research indicates safety, and treating depressed patients with acute angina or following myocardial infarction may reduce cardiac events

No dose adjustment for renal impairment. Not removed by hemodialysis

Lower dose by half or give less frequently for hepatic impairment

FIGURE 2.11. Dosing and interaction information for fluoxetine.

Sertraline

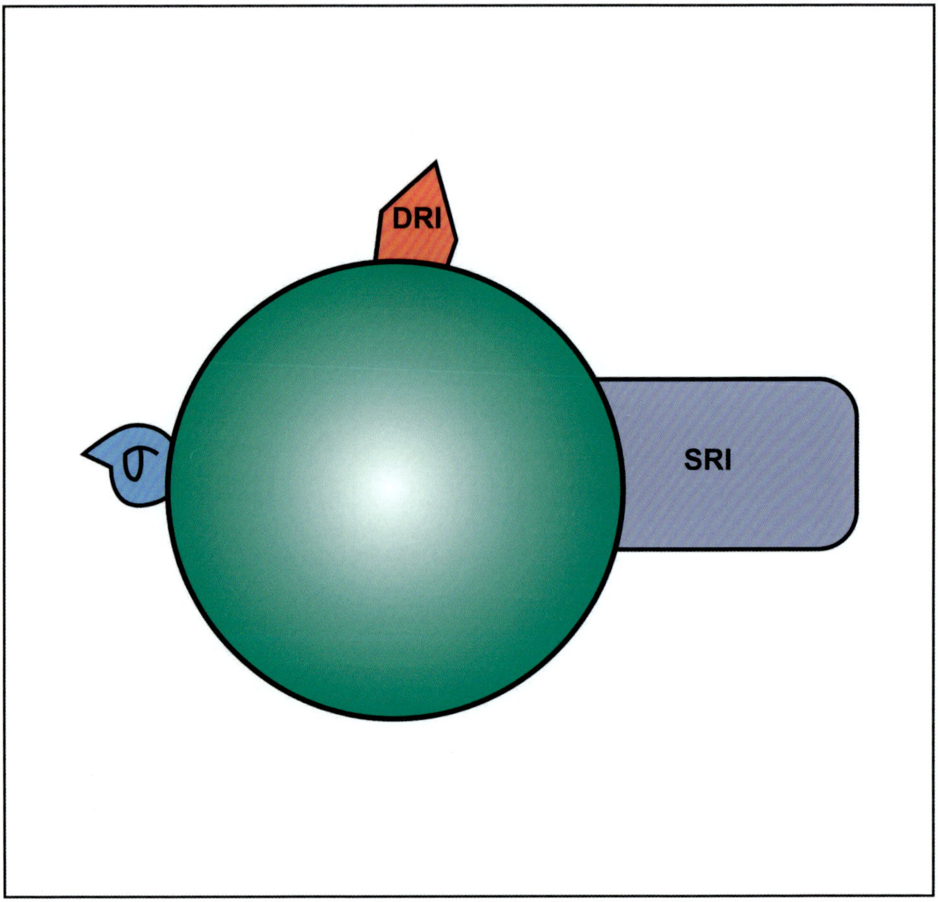

FIGURE 2.12. Sertraline is unique in that it binds to sigma-1 receptors as well as the dopamine transporter (DAT), acting as a dopamine reuptake inhibitor (DRI) in addition to its SRI properties. While sigma-1 actions are not well understood, they may contribute to anxiolytic effects and may be useful in psychotic depression. The actions at DAT may be weak, but perhaps only a small amount of DAT inhibition is enough to cause improvement of certain depressive symptoms when utilized in conjunction with SERT (serotonin transporter) inhibition. Sertraline may be added to bupropion, another DAT inhibitor, increasing that property and aiding in alleviation of depressive symptoms.

Sertraline: Tips and Pearls

Dosing

Formulation:
25, 50 mg scored, 100 mg tablets; 20 mg/mL – 60 mL bottles liquid

Dosage Range:
50-200 mg/day

Approved For:
Major depressive disorder, premenstrual dysphoric disorder, post-traumatic stress disorder, obsessive compulsive disorder, panic disorder, social anxiety disorder

Pearls

May be first-line choice for atypical depression. May be type of "dual-action" agent with 5HT and DA reuptake inhibition

Use with caution in children. Watch for induction of mania or suicidal ideation. Approved for use in children with OCD

Pregnancy risk category C (some animal studies show adverse effects, no controlled studies in humans)

Side effects I

Weight Gain

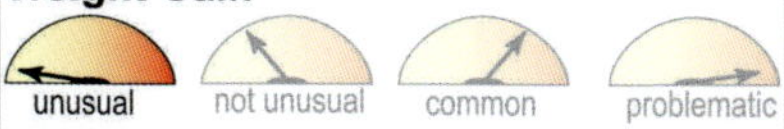

Sedation

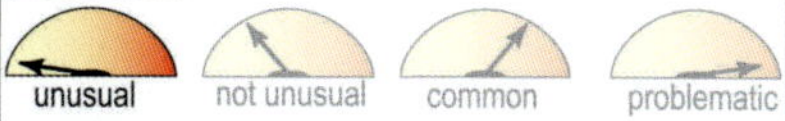

Rare seizures, induction of mania and suicidality

Side effects II

Do not use with MAOIs, thioridazine, pimozide, disulfiram (liquid)

Proven cardiovascular safety in depressed patients with myocardial infarction or angina

No dose adjustment for renal impairment. Not removed by hemodialysis

Lower dose by half or give less frequently for hepatic impairment

FIGURE 2.13. Dosing and interaction information for sertraline.

Paroxetine

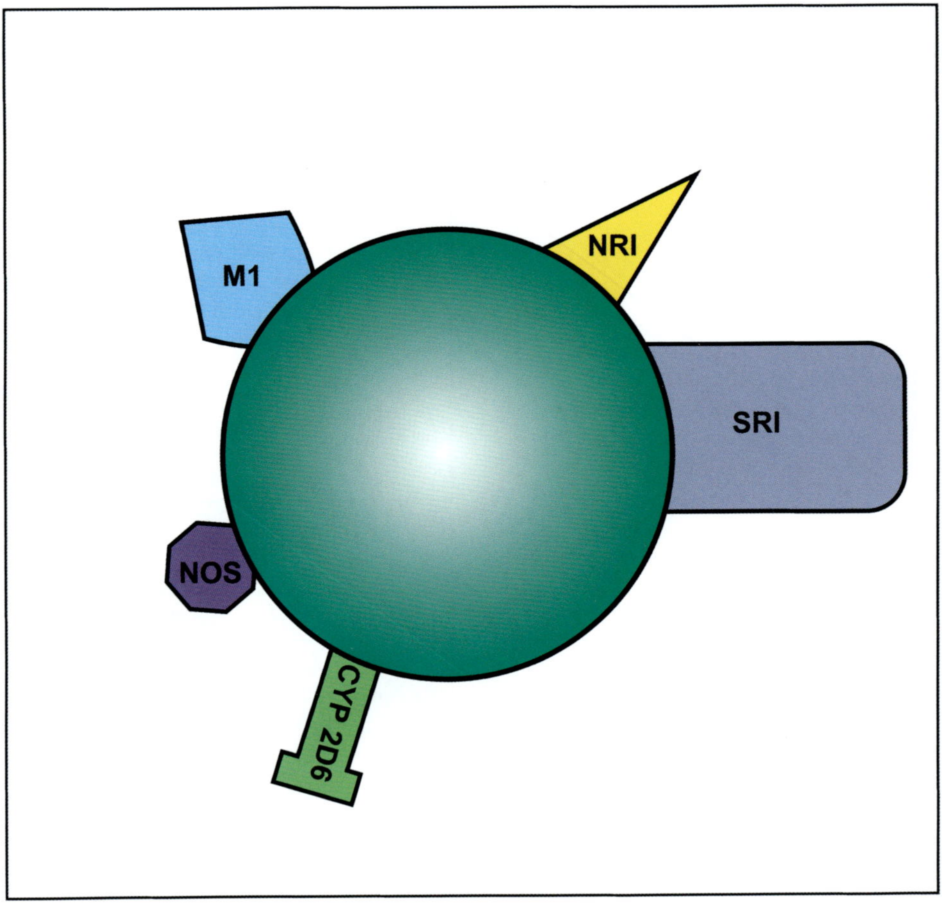

FIGURE 2.14. Paroxetine is often preferred in the treatment of depression for patients with anxiety symptoms. This may be due to paroxetine's anticholinergic effects (M1 muscarinic antagonism). In addition to this and SRI (serotonin reuptake inhibition) properties, paroxetine has weak NET (norepinephrine transporter) inhibition properties, thus acting as a norepinephrine reuptake inhibitor (NRI) with potent inhibitory actions at CYP450 2D6. Paroxetine is a substrate as well as an inhibitor of 2D6, which can lead to a rapid decline in its plasma drug levels when paroxetine is discontinued, contributing to the withdrawal symptoms experienced upon sudden discontinuation. Inhibition of NOS (nitric oxide synthetase) may contribute to sexual dysfunction side effects.

Paroxetine: Tips and Pearls

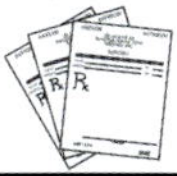

Dosing

Formulation:
10, 20 mg scored, 30 and 40 mg tablets. CR 12.5, 25 mg. Liquid 10 mg/5-250 ml bottle

Dosage Range:
20-50 mg; 25-62.5 mg CR

Approved For:
Major depressive disorder, obsessive compulsive disorder, posttraumatic stress disorder, social anxiety disorder, premenstrual dysphoric disorder, panic disorder, generalized anxiety disorder

Side effects I

Weight Gain

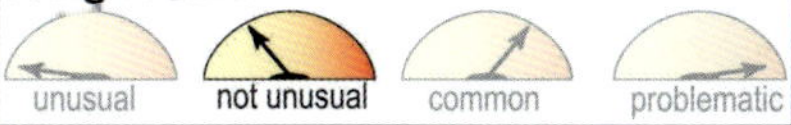

Sedation

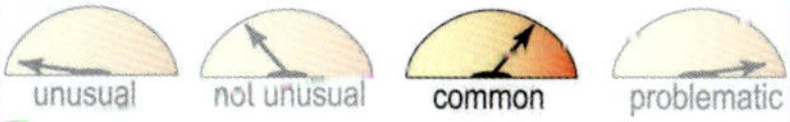

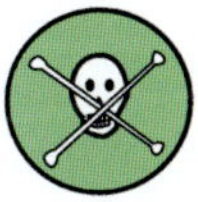

Rare seizures, induction of mania and suicidality

Pearls

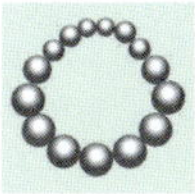

Often preferred treatment for anxious depression and major depression with comorbid anxiety disorders. Withdrawal effects may be more likely than with other SSRIs when discontinued. Mild anticholinergic actions which can enhance rapid onset of efficacy but also cause mild anticholinergic side effects

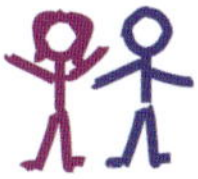

Use with caution in children. Watch for induction of mania or suicidal ideation

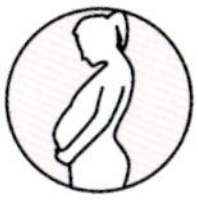

Pregnancy risk category D (positive evidence of risk to human fetus; potential benefits may still justify its use during pregnancy)

Side effects II

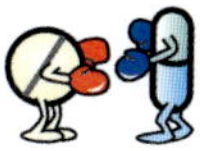

Via CYP450 2D6 inhibition, may increase concentrations of other drugs. May increase anticholinergic effects of other drugs. Do not use with MAOIs, thioridazine, pimozide

Preliminary research suggests that it is safe for patients with cardiac impairment

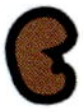

Lower dose for renal impairment; maximum 40 mg/day

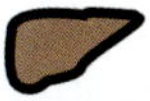

Lower dose for hepatic impairment; maximum 40 mg/day

FIGURE 2.15. Dosing and interaction information for paroxetine.

Fluvoxamine

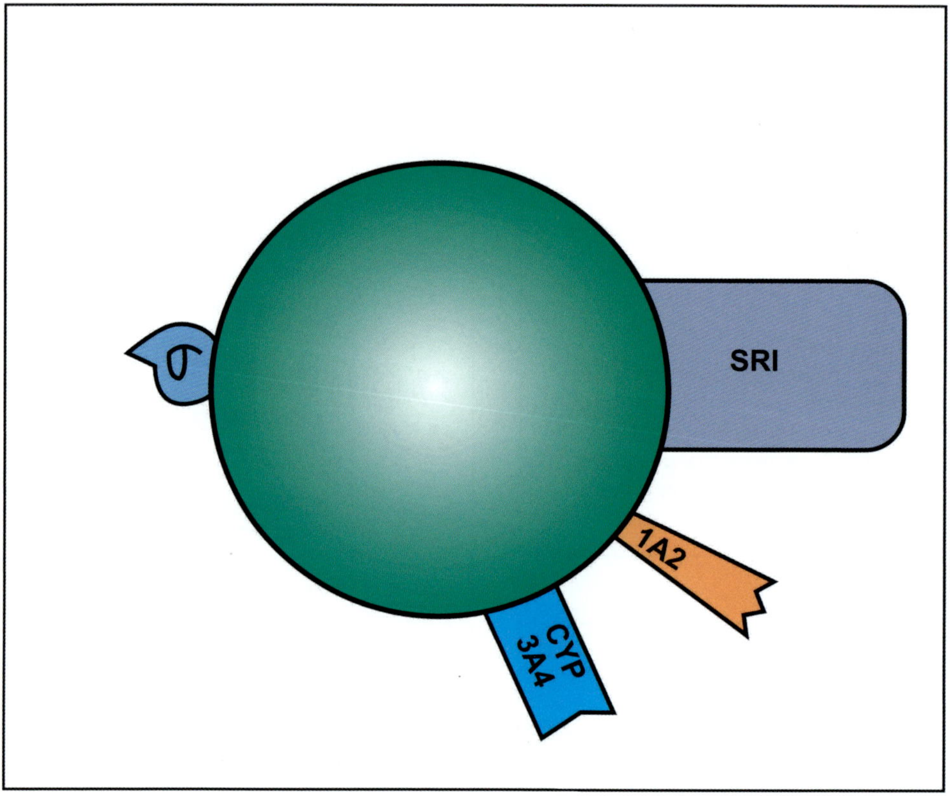

FIGURE 2.16. Fluvoxamine has potentially important secondary actions at sigma-1 receptors. This action is more potent for fluvoxamine than sertraline, with fluvoxamine's properties thought to be agonistic at sigma-1 receptors, contributing to its efficacy as an anxiolytic. Additionally, fluvoxamine has shown therapeutic effect as a treatment option in psychotic and delusional depression. Currently available as a controlled-release formulation, once-a-day administration is possible and favored, with clinical trials reporting robust remission rates in obsessive compulsive disorder and anxiety disorder. Fluvoxamine is also available in immediate-release formulation, but due to shorter half-life, this requires twice-daily administration. Fluvoxamine was one of the first antidepressants marketed worldwide, though it was never approved for depression in the U.S. (currently used more often in the treatment of OCD and anxiety). It is a potent inhibitor of CYP450 1A2 and 3A4.

Fluvoxamine: Tips and Pearls

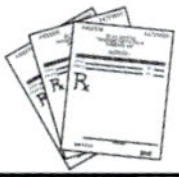

Dosing

Formulation:
25, 50, 100 mg scored tablets;
100 and 150 mg CR capsules

Dosage Range:
100-200 mg/day for depression
100-300 mg/day for OCD

Approved For:
Obsessive compulsive disorder

Pearls

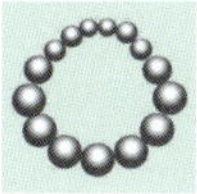

Recently released in CR formulation. Often preferred treatment for anxious depression and major depressive disorder with comorbid anxiety disorders. Actions at sigma 1 receptors may explain advantage for psychotic and delusional depression. May also explain rapid onset effects in anxiety and insomnia

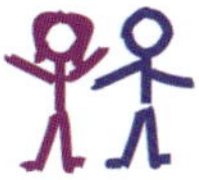

Use with caution in children. Watch for induction of mania or suicidal ideation. Approved for ages 8-17 for OCD

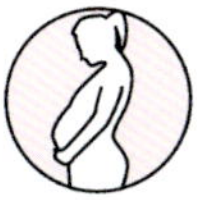

Pregnancy risk category C (some animal studies show adverse effects, no controlled studies in humans)

Side effects I

Weight Gain

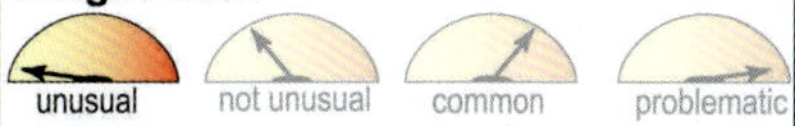

Sedation

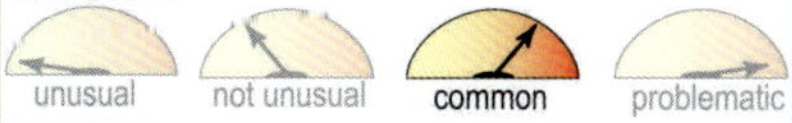

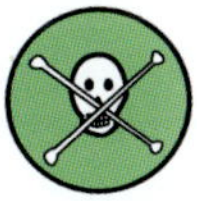

Rare seizures, induction of mania and suicidality

Side effects II

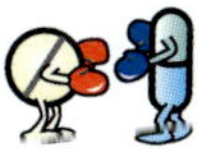

Via CYP450 1A2 and 3A4 inhibition, may increase concentrations of other drugs. Do not use with MAOIs, thioridazine, pimozide

Preliminary research suggests it is safe for patients with cardiac impairment

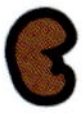

No dose adjustment for renal impairment

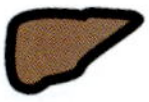

Lower dose or give less frequently for hepatic impairment. Use slower titration

FIGURE 2.17. Dosing and interaction information for fluvoxamine.

Citalopram

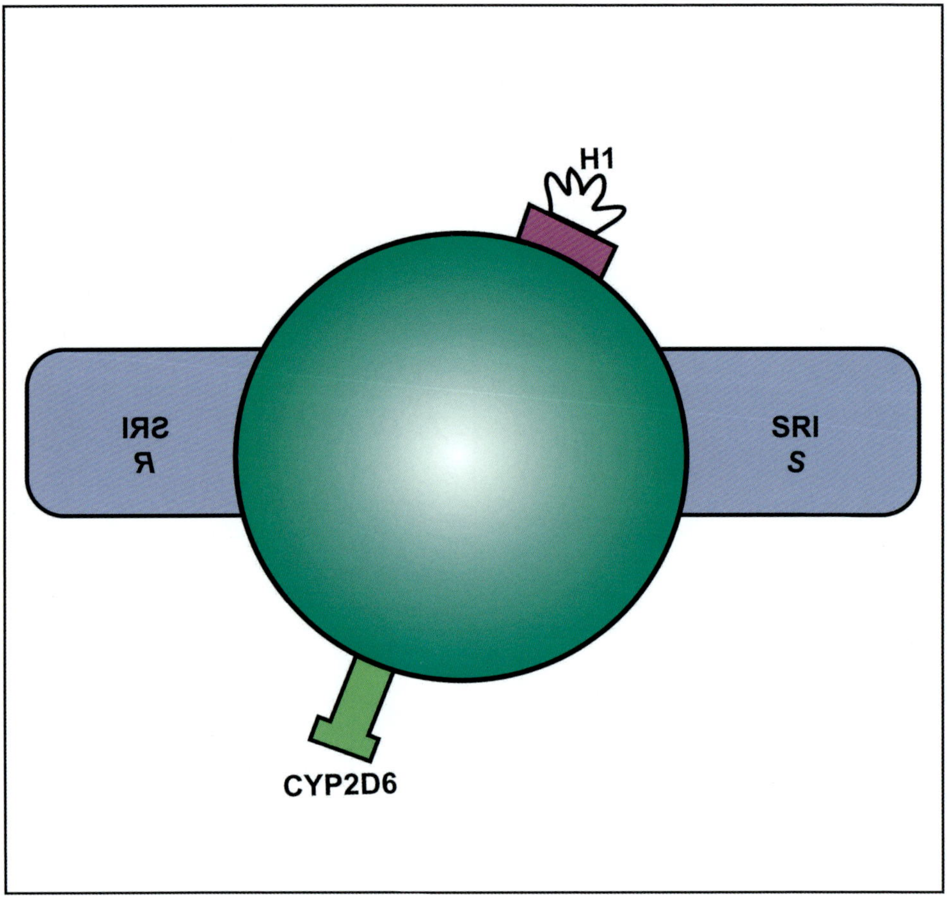

FIGURE 2.18. Citalopram consists of two enantiomers, R and S. Taken together, this agent is known as racemic citalopram, with mild antihistamine and 2D6 inhibitory properties residing in the R enantiomer. Citalopram is generally a well-tolerated SSRI and is useful in treating elderly patients with depression. However, citalopram may be somewhat inconsistent in therapeutic action at its lowest dose, potentially requiring a dose increase to optimize treatment response. This may be due to a recent finding that the R enantiomer may be active at SERT, interfering with the ability of the S enantiomer to inhibit SERT. This interference could lead to reduced inhibition of SERT, reduced synaptic serotonin and possibly reduced therapeutic action.

Citalopram: Tips and Pearls

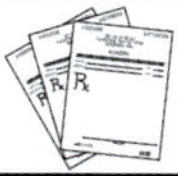

Dosing

Formulation:
10 mg, 20 and 40 mg scored tablets

Dosage Range:
20-40 mg/day

Approved For:
Depression

Pearls

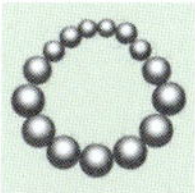

May be better tolerated than other antidepressants but less well tolerated than escitalopram

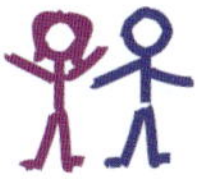

Use with caution in children. Watch for induction of mania or suicidal ideation

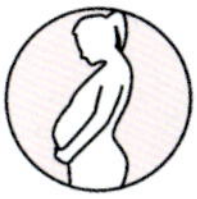

Pregnancy risk category C (some animal studies show adverse effects, no controlled studies in humans)

Side effects I

Weight Gain

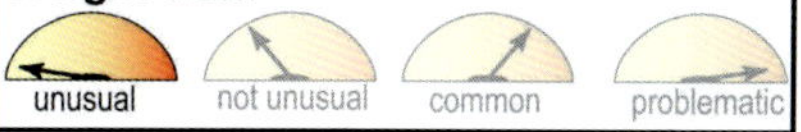

Weight Gain

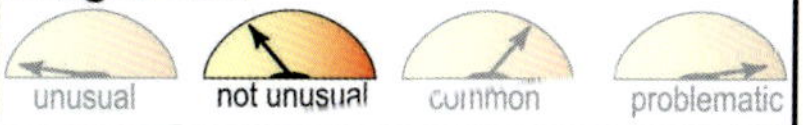

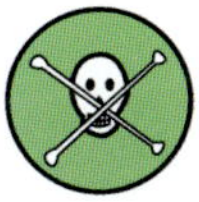

Rare seizures, induction of mania and suicidality

Side effects II

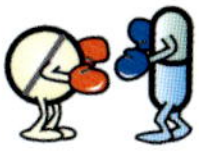

Via CYP450 2D6 inhibition, may increase concentrations of other drugs. Do not use with MAOIs, thioridazine

Should not be used in patients with congenital long QT syndrome; patients with congestive heart failure, bradyarrhythmias, or predisposition to hypokalemia or hypomagnesemia because of concomitant illness or drugs, are at higher risk of developing Torsade de Pointes

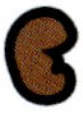

No dose adjustment in patients with mild to moderate renal impairment. Use with caution

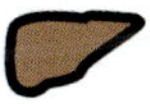

Recommended dose 20 mg/day for hepatic impairment. May use 40 mg/day in non-responders. Use with caution

FIGURE 2.19. Dosing and interaction information for citalopram.

Escitalopram

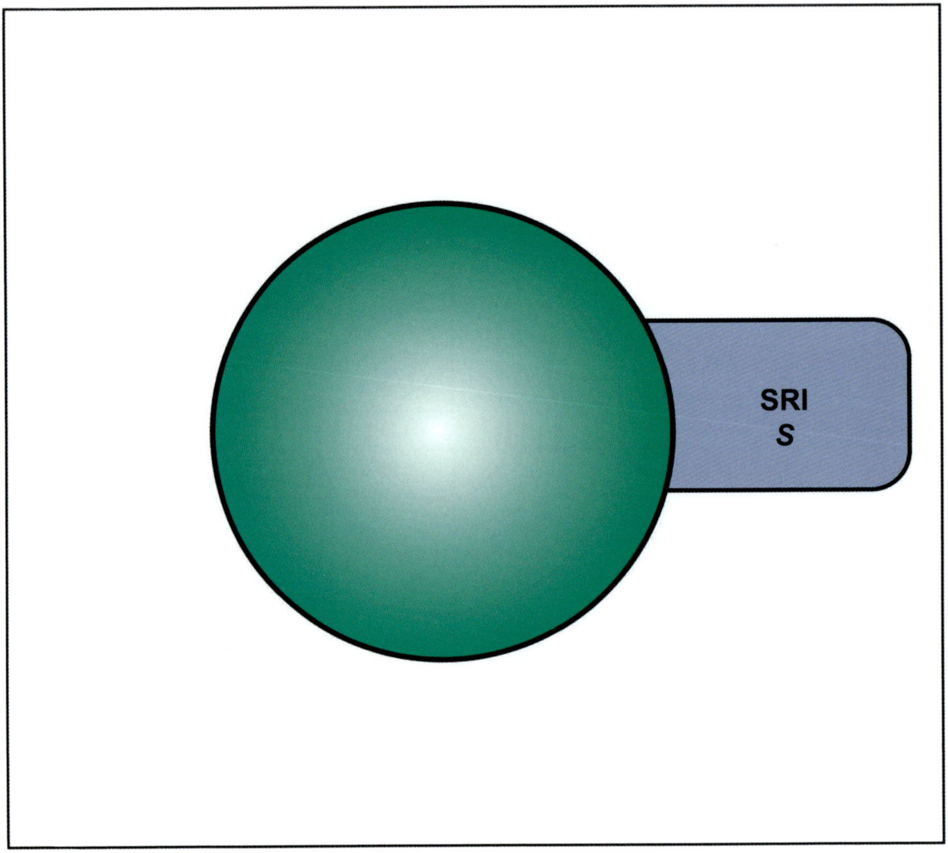

FIGURE 2.20. Escitalopram is, in essence, citalopram with the R enantiomer removed. In this case, the pure active SERT properties of the S enantiomer are the cause of its antidepressant properties. By removing the R enantiomer, this also removes the antihistaminic and CYP450 2D6 inhibitory properties of citalopram. Additionally, by removing the R enantiomer, which can interfere with SERT, the lowest dose of escitalopram may be more effective. Escitalopram is known as one of the better-tolerated SSRIs with the fewest CYP450-mediated drug interactions, though it is comparatively expensive, as no generic is yet available.

Escitalopram: Tips and Pearls

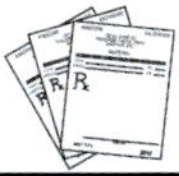

Dosing

Formulation:
10 and 20 mg tablets

Dosage Range:
10-20 mg/day. Oral solution 5 mg/5 mL

Approved For:
Major depressive disorder, generalized anxiety disorder

Pearls

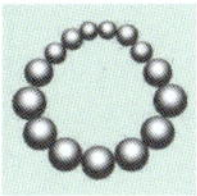

May be among best-tolerated antidepressants. R citalopram may interfere with binding of S citalopram at SERT. Commonly used with augmenting agents, as it has least interaction at CYP450 2D6 and 3A4, causing fewer pharmacokinetically mediated drug interactions

Use with caution in children. Watch for induction of mania or suicidal ideation

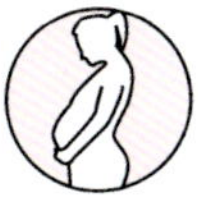

Pregnancy risk category C (some animal studies show adverse effects, no controlled studies in humans)

Side effects I

Weight Gain

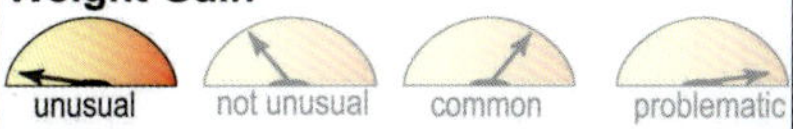

Sedation

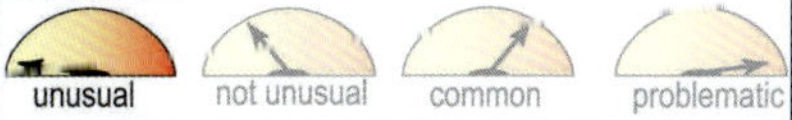

Rare seizures, induction of mania and suicidality

Side effects II

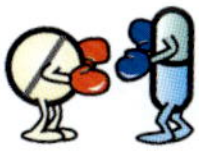

Few known adverse drug interactions. Do not use with MAOIs

Not well evaluated in patients with cardiac impairment

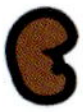

Start with 10 mg/day for renal impairment

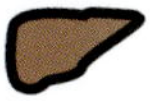

Recommended dose 10 mg/day for hepatic impairment

FIGURE 2.21. Dosing and interaction information for escitalopram.

Molecular Actions of SNRIs:

Part 1, Primary Actions on Serotonin and Norepinephrine Throughout the Brain

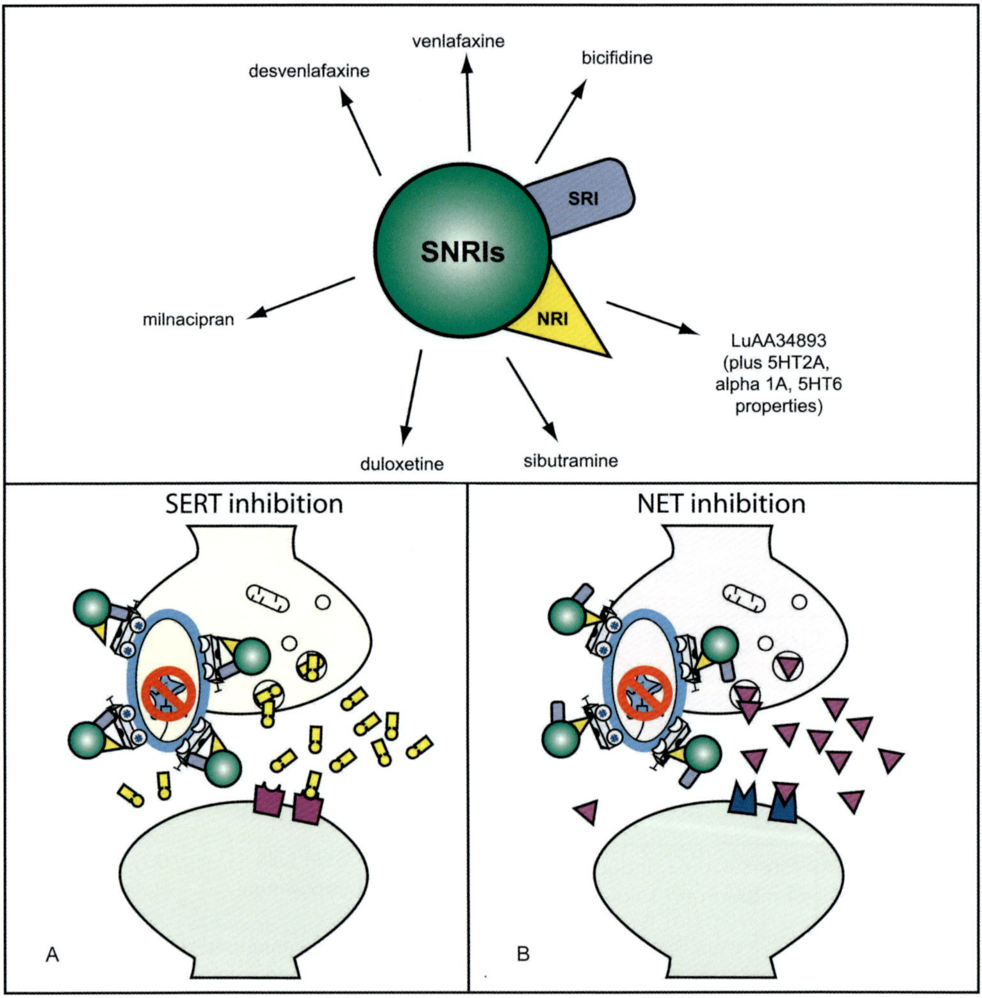

FIGURE 2.22. SNRI dual action properties (shown at top). The SRI (serotonin reuptake inhibition) property of SNRIs plugs into SERT (serotonin transporter), resulting in an increase of synaptic 5HT and an antidepressant effect (A). The NRI (norepinephrine reuptake inhibition) property of SNRIs inserts into the norepinephrine transporter (NET), thereby allowing increased amounts of NE into the synapse and again, an antidepressant effect (B).

Molecular Actions of SNRIs:
Part 2, Secondary Actions on Dopamine in Prefrontal Cortex

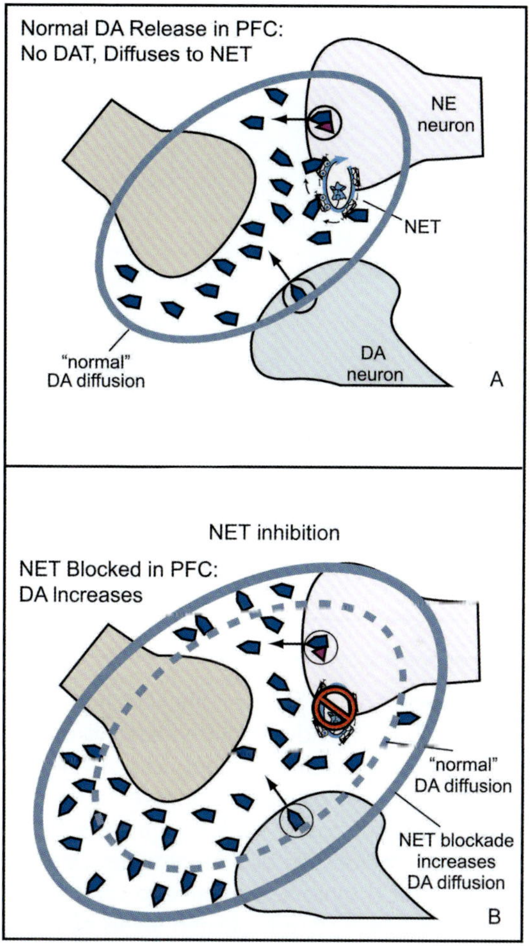

FIGURE 2.23. Dopamine is normally inactivated in the prefrontal cortex (PFC) by the NET (norepinephrine transporter is shown above). That is, the DA neurons in PFC largely lack DA transporters (see lack of DATs on the DA neurons above), so DA diffuses after release until it reaches a NET on a NE neuron (A). NETs actually have higher affinity for DA than they do for NE! Thus, in PFC, NETs inactivate both NE and DA. The consequence of this is that when NET is blocked, both NE and DA increase (B) (see Fig. 2.22B).

Venlafaxine

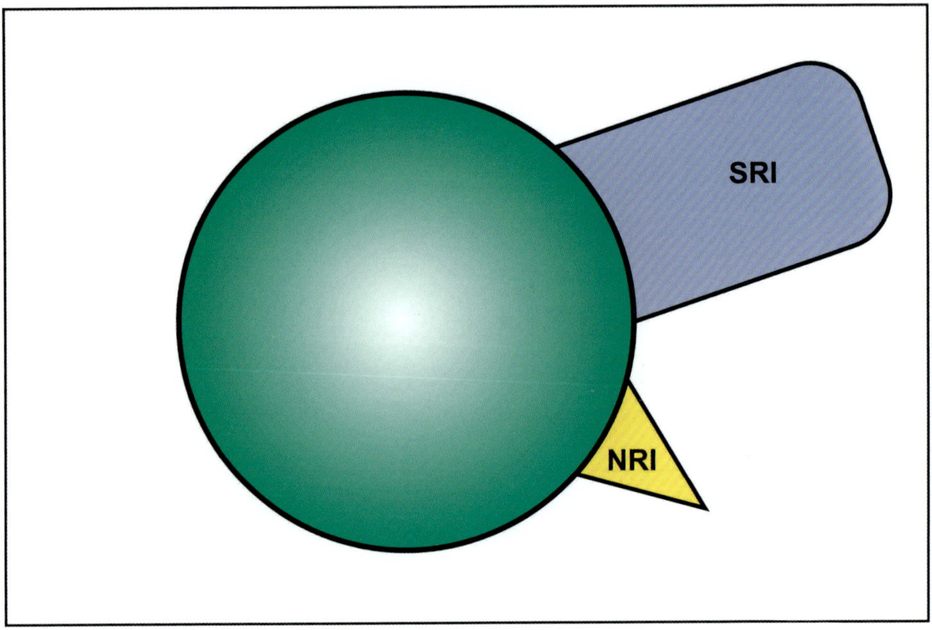

FIGURE 2.24. Venlafaxine was the first SNRI on the U.S. market, and has become one of the most frequently prescribed individual antidepressants on the market, particularly among psychiatrists. Venlafaxine has differing degrees of inhibition of norepinephrine reuptake depending on the dose, whereas serotonin reuptake inhibition is moderately potent and present at all approved doses. Venlafaxine is a substrate for CYP450 2D6, which converts it to the active metabolite desvenlafaxine. Desvenlafaxine has greater norepinephrine transporter (NET) inhibition relative to serotonin transporter (SERT) inhibition. After venlafaxine is administered, plasma levels of venlafaxine are normally around half that of desvenlafaxine. If a CYP450 2D6 inhibitor is taken concurrently, this may shift the plasma levels more toward venlafaxine, reducing the amount of NET inhibition. This variability of plasma levels may also accompany CYP450 2D6 genetic polymorphisms, with poor metabolizers shifting the plasma concentration more toward venlafaxine, which may result in a reduction of NET inhibition. Dose titration of venlafaxine or administration of desvenlafaxine itself (see Figs. 2.26 and 2.27) may solve this problem. Venlafaxine may have withdrawal reactions, especially after sudden discontinuation. The extended release formulation is much better tolerated than the immediate release formulation.

Venlafaxine: Tips and Pearls

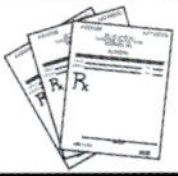

Dosing

Formulation:
Capsule (ER) 37.5, 75 and 150 mg. Tablets 25, 37.5, 50, 75 and 100 mg scored

Dosage Range:
150-225 mg/day for generalized anxiety disorder, 75-225 mg/day for depression once daily (extended release) or divided into 2-3 doses (immediate release)

Approved For:
Depression, generalized anxiety disorder, social anxiety disorder, panic disorder

Pearls

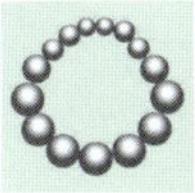

May be useful for patients with treatment-resistant depression or in combination with other antidepressants for treatment-refractory cases. Greater potency for serotonin reuptake blockade than norepinephrine reuptake blockade. Preliminary studies suggest efficacy in neuropathic pain and fibromyalgia

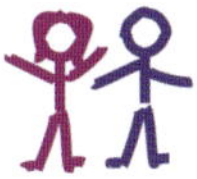

Use with caution in children. Watch for induction of mania or suicidal ideation

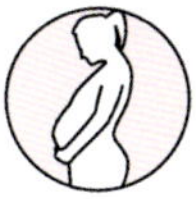

Pregnancy risk category C (some animal studies show adverse effects, no controlled studies in humans)

Side effects I

Weight Gain

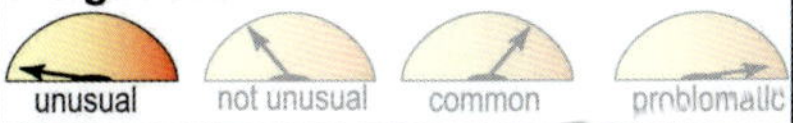

Sedation

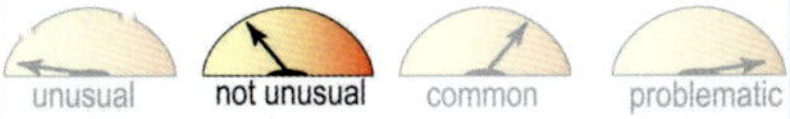

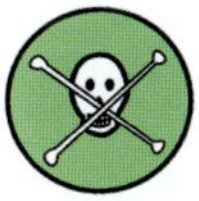

Rare seizures, induction of mania and suicidality

Side effects II

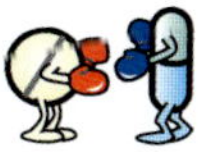

Few known adverse drug interactions. Do not use with MAOIs

Use with caution in patients with cardiovascular disease

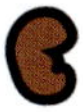

Lower dose by 25-50% for renal impairment. Patients on dialysis shouldn't receive subsequent dose until dialysis is completed

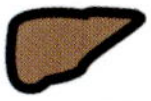

Lower dose by 50% for hepatic impairment

FIGURE 2.25. Dosing and interaction information for venlafaxine.

Desvenlafaxine (Active Metabolite of Venlafaxine)

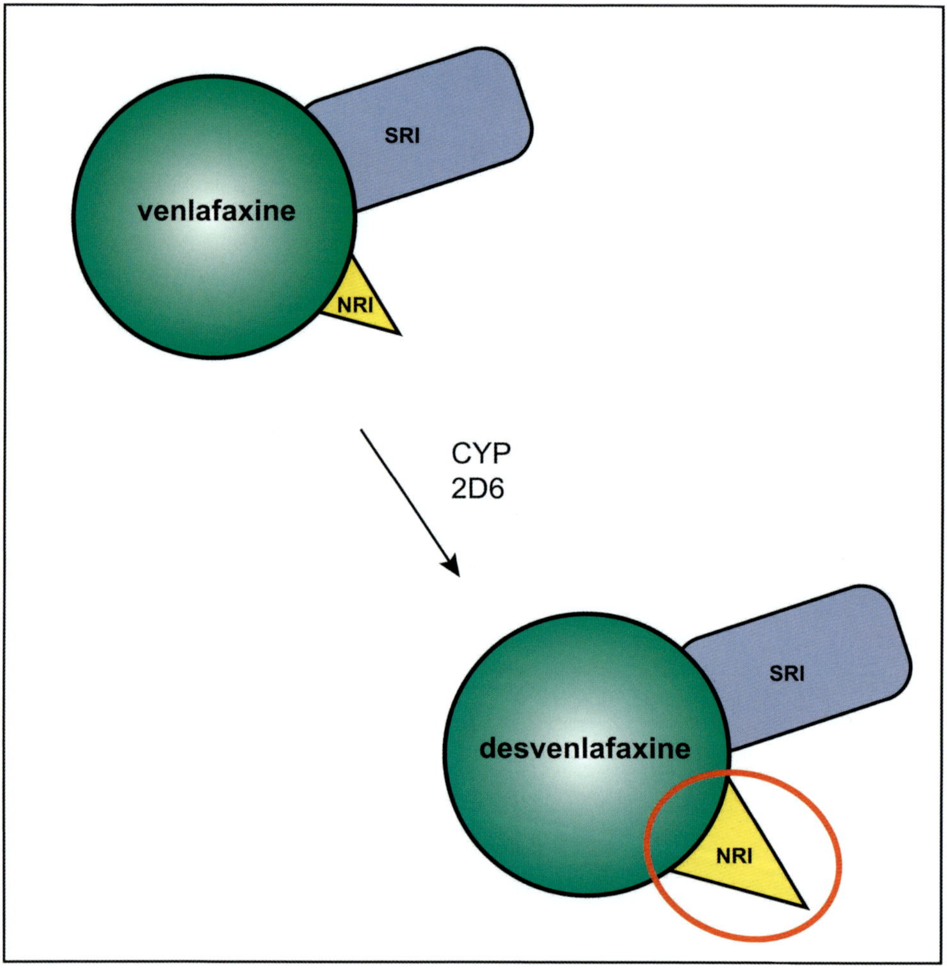

FIGURE 2.26. Desvenlafaxine has greater NET inhibition than SERT inhibition compared to venlafaxine. Since desvenlafaxine is not a substrate of CYP450 enzymes including 2D6, plasma levels should be more consistent than with venlafaxine. Additionally, desvenlafaxine is not affected by genetic polymorphisms of CYP450. Thus, the relative amount of NET versus SERT should also be more consistent, and greater at comparable doses. Desvenlafaxine has been tested for treatment of vasomotor symptoms associated with perimenopause, with positive results.

Desvenlafaxine: Tips and Pearls

Dosing

Formulation:
50 and 100 mg tablets

Dosage Range:
50 mg once daily. Clinical studies indicate 50-400 mg/day effective; greater dose does not add proven benefits

Approved For:
Major depressive disorder

Pearls

Approved at once-daily dose. Titration may not be necessary in first-line use. Discontinuation rate due to side effects similar to placebo. Off-label use for vasomotor symptoms in perimenopausal women who do not wish to take estrogen can be considered (caution for cardiovascular side effects)

Use with caution in children. Watch for induction of mania or suicidal ideation

Pregnancy risk category C (some animal studies show adverse effects, no controlled studies in humans)

Side effects I

Weight Gain
unusual · not unusual · common · problematic

Sedation
unusual · not unusual · common · problematic

Seizures may occur. Use with caution. Watch for suicidal ideations and mania induction

Side effects II

Do not use with MAOIs

Use with caution in patients with cardiovascular disease

Dose should not exceed 50 mg/day in moderate cases of renal impairment

Doses higher than 50 mg/day not recommended for hepatic impairment. Use with caution

FIGURE 2.27. Dosing and interaction information for desvenlafaxine.

Duloxetine

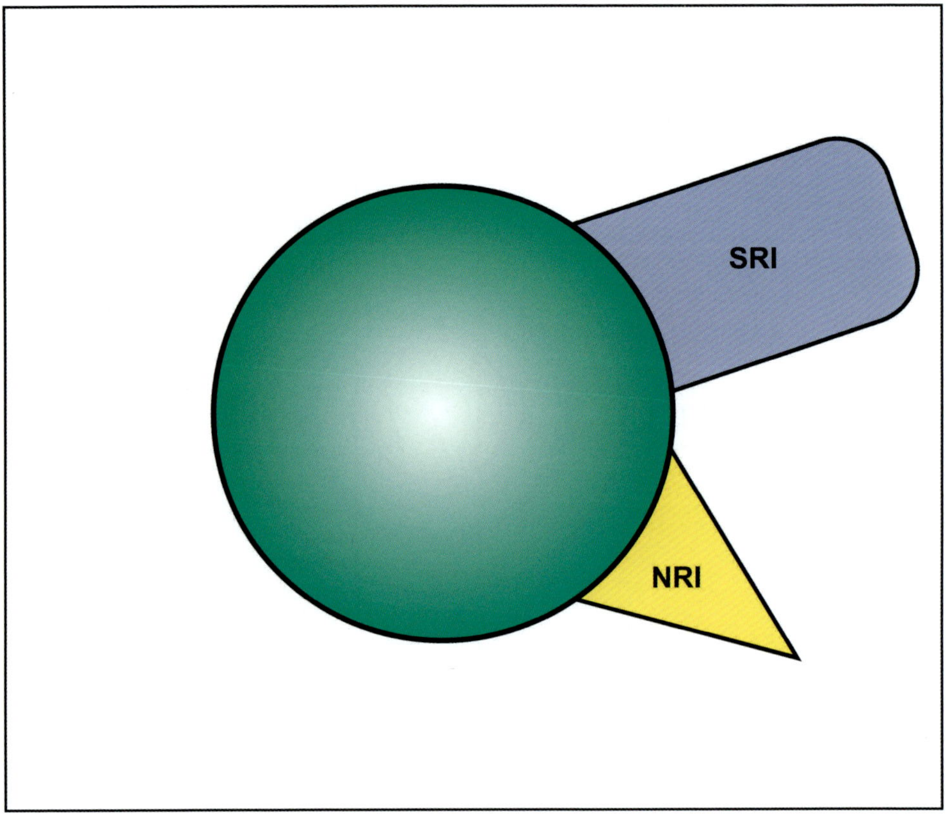

FIGURE 2.28. Duloxetine is the first SNRI approved for treatment of painful neuropathy (diabetic peripheral neuropathic pain), in addition to treating major depression and generalized anxiety disorder. This agent appears to be useful in treating the painful physical symptoms associated with a major depressive episode, as well as treating geriatric depression, which is often associated with cognitive dysfunction. Duloxetine has shown efficacy in treating the pain associated with fibromyalgia and may also be useful for cognitive symptoms in fibromyalgia. Improvement of cognition in various disorders may be due to NET inhibition in prefrontal cortex (see Fig. 2.23). Duloxetine is a CYP450 2D6 inhibitor, which may result in various drug interactions that should be monitored. Duloxetine may be administered once daily, though in some difficult to treat patients, higher doses may be utilized, which may be dosed twice daily.

Duloxetine: Tips and Pearls

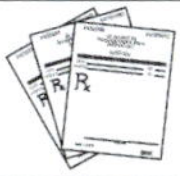

Dosing

Formulation:
20,30 and 60 mg capsules

Dosage Range:
40-60 mg/day in 1-2 doses for depression. 60 mg/day once/day for DPNP. 40 mg 2x/day for stress urinary incontinence (in Europe)

Approved For:
Major depressive disorder, diabetic peripheral neuropathic pain, fibromyalgia, acute and chronic generalized anxiety disorder, chronic musculoskeletal pain

Pearls

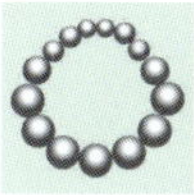

May have particular efficacy for painful symptoms of depression. Approved in many countries for stress urinary incontinence. Approval pending for fibromyalgia. May be useful for pain and "fibro-fog" (cognition) in fibromyalgia

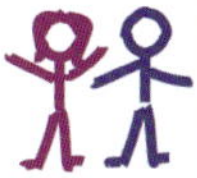

Use with caution in children. Watch for induction of mania or suicidal ideation

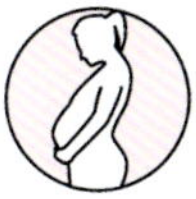

Pregnancy risk category C (some animal studies show adverse effects, no controlled studies in humans)

Side effects I

Weight Gain

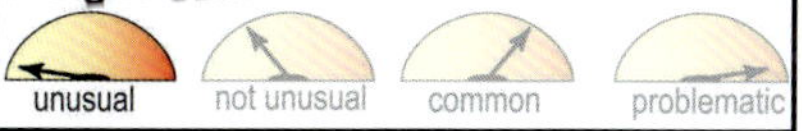

Sedation

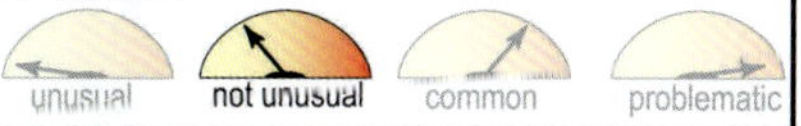

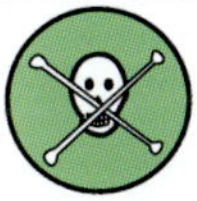

Rare seizures, induction of mania and suicidality

Side effects II

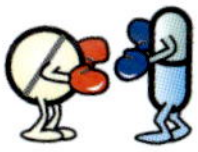

Inhibitors of CYP450 2D6 may increase plasma levels and require dosage reduction of duloxetine. Do not use with MAOIs, thioridazine

Use with caution in patient with cardiac impairment; may raise blood pressure

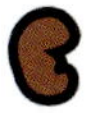

Not recommended for use in patients with end-stage renal disease

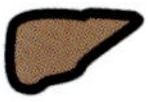

Not to be used in patients with any hepatic insufficiencies. Do not use in patients who use or abuse alcohol

FIGURE 2.29. Dosing and interaction information for duloxetine.

Milnacipran

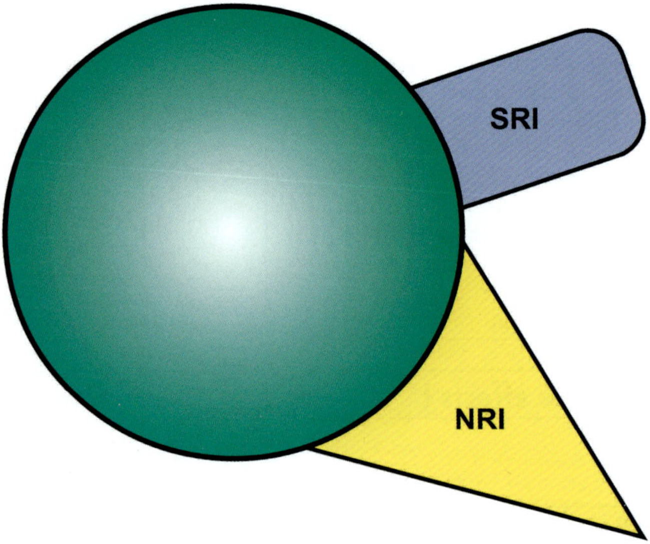

FIGURE 2.30. Milnacipran is somewhat different than other SNRIs in that it has the strongest relative actions at NET compared to SERT among the four approved SNRIs. Some data even suggest that its actions at NET are stronger than those at SERT, while the other SNRIs are generally the opposite. Data suggest that milnacipran may have efficacy both for pain and cognitive symptoms in fibromyalgia. Milnacipran is approved for the treatment of depression in several countries outside the US, and approval for fibromyalgia is pending worldwide. Milnacipran may be more energizing and activating than some other SNRIs due to its relatively potent noradrenergic actions, and may cause more sweating and urinary hesitancy. Milnacipran is generally given twice daily due to its short half-life.

Milnacipran: Tips and Pearls

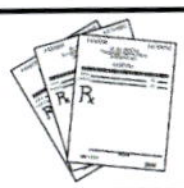

Dosing

Formulation:
12.5, 25, 50, 100 mg tablet (U.S.). 25 and 50 mg capsules (European and other worldwide markets). 15, 25 and 50 mg capsules (Japan)

Dosage Range:
30-200 mg/day in 2 doses

Approved For:
Commonly prescribed for major depressive disorder, and fibromyalgia

Pearls

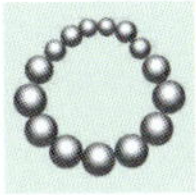

Relatively greater potency for NE reuptake blockade than 5HT reuptake blockade compared to other SNRIs. Onset of action in fibromyalgia may be faster than depression. Potent noradrenergic actions may account for higher incidence of sweating and urinary hesitancy as well as theoretical advantages for cognitive symptoms in fibromyalgia ("fibrofog")

Use with caution in children. Watch for induction of mania or suicidal ideation

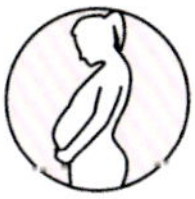

Pregnancy risk category C (some animal studies show adverse effects, no controlled studies in humans)

Side effects I

Weight Gain

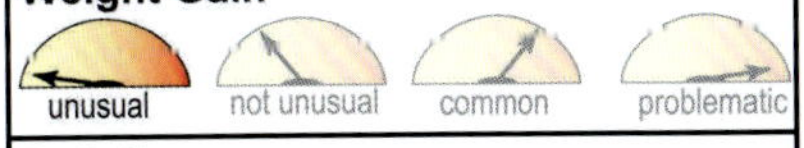

Sedation

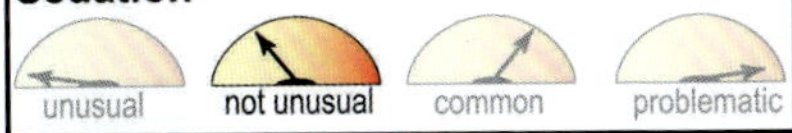

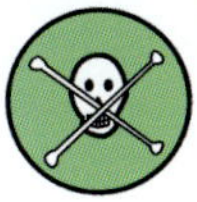

Rare seizures, induction of mania and suicidality

Side effects II

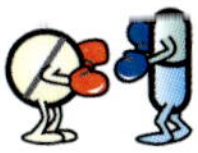

Few known adverse pharmacokinetic drug interactions. Do not use with MAOIs

Use with caution in patients with cardiac impairment

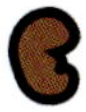

Should receive lower doses in relation to degree of renal impairment

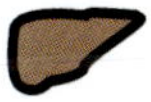

No dose adjustment necessary for hepatic impairment

FIGURE 2.31. Dosing and interaction information for milnacipran.

Stahl's Illustrated | Chapter 3

Norepinephrine and Dopamine Reuptake Inhibitors (NDRIs) and Selective Norepinephrine Reuptake Inhibitors (NRIs)

This chapter reviews the antidepressant drugs that are combined norepinephrine dopamine reuptake inhibitors (NDRIs) and selective norepinephrine reuptake inhibitors (NRIs), and that are currently available to clinicians. NDRIs are considered first-line treatment, and NRIs are often second-line. Each drug in these classes is reviewed. The aim of this chapter is to familiarize the reader with these options for treating depression.

Symbols Used in this Chapter			
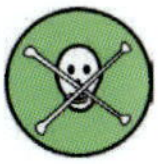	Life-threatening or Dangerous Side Effects	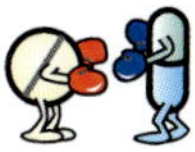	Drug Interactions
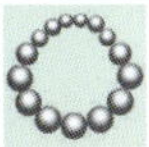	Tips and Pearls		Cardiac Impairment
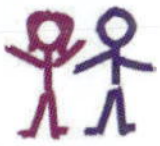	Children and Adolescents	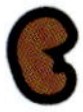	Renal Impairment
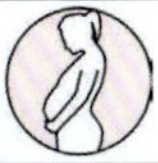	Pregnancy	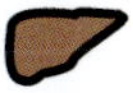	Hepatic Impairment

NDRI and NRI Antidepressants

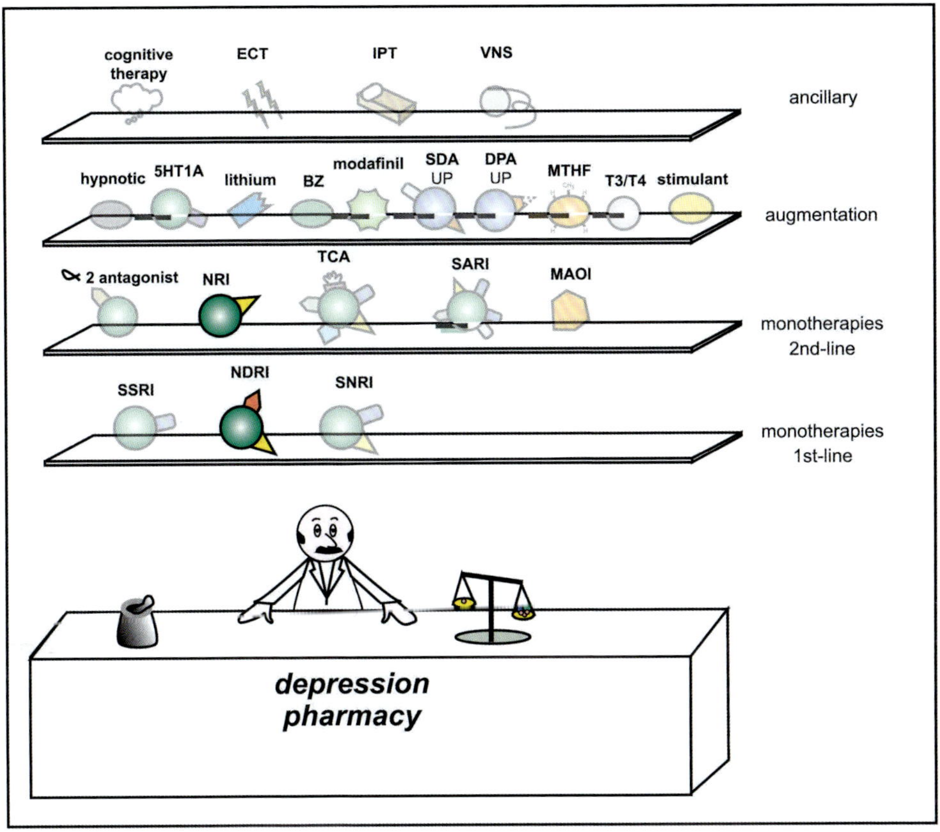

FIGURE 3.1. NDRIs are on the first-line treatment shelf, whereas NRIs are second-line monotherapies.

SSRI: selective serotonin reuptake inhibitors. NDRI: norepinephrine dopamine reuptake inhibitors. SNRI: serotonin norepinephrine reuptake inhibitors. SDA: serotonin dopamine antagonists. α 2 antagonist: alpha 2 antagonists. NRI: selective norepinephrine reuptake inhibitors. TCA: tricyclic antidepressants. SARI: serotonin 2A antagonist/ reuptake inhibitors. MAOI: monoamine oxidase inhibitors. 5HT1A: serotonin 1A partial agonists. BZ: benzodiazepines. DPA: dopamine partial agonists. MTHF: L-5-methyltetrahydrofolate. T3/T4: thyroid hormone. ECT: electroconvulsive therapy. IPT: interpersonal therapy. VNS: vagus nerve stimulation.

Comparing the Molecular Actions of NDRIs and Selective NRIs

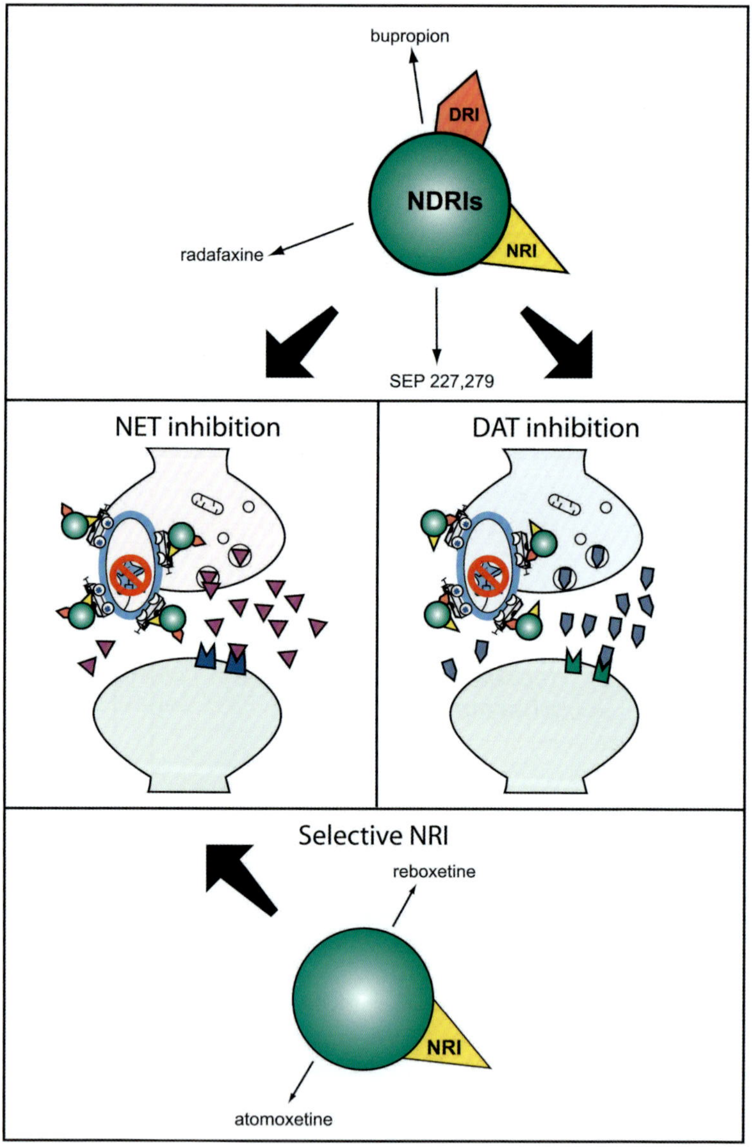

FIGURE 3.2. NDRIs inhibit both the norepinephrine transporter (NET) and the dopamine transporter (DAT), whereas selective NRIs inhibit only NET.

Comparing the Regional Effects of NDRIs and NRIs

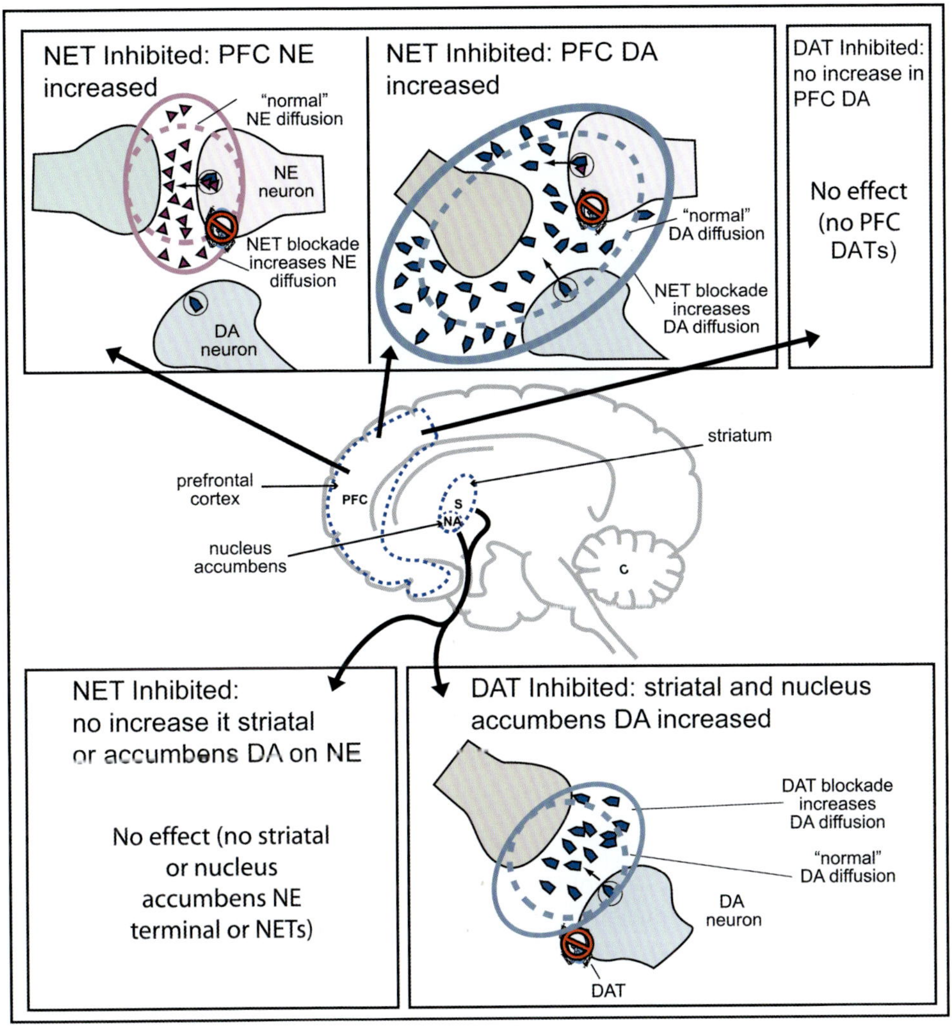

FIGURE 3.3. Both NDRIs and NRIs raise both NE and DA in the prefrontal cortex due to inhibition of NETs there (top figures). NDRIs, however, show regionally differential actions in the striatum and nucleus accumbens, raising DA but not NE, due to inhibition of DATs there. On the other hand, NRIs increase neither NE nor DA in the striatum and nucleus accumbens, due to the lack of NETs there.

PFC: prefrontal cortex, NA: nucleus accumbens, S: striatum

Bupropion

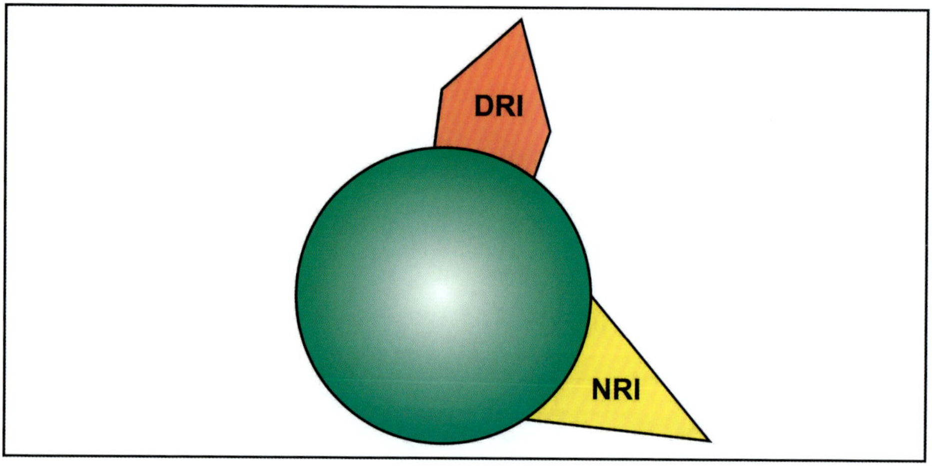

FIGURE 3.4. Bupropion has less potent NET and DAT blocking properties than SSRIs and SNRIs generally have for SERT blockade. This implies either that NET and DAT inhibition are insufficient explanations of bupropion's antidepressant actions, or that lesser amounts of NET and DAT inhibition are necessary to be an antidepressant than SERT inhibition. The latter possibility is supported by observations that much less NET inhibition than SERT inhibition occurs with SNRI use (see previous chapter) and that high degrees of DAT inhibition include abusable stimulants such as amphetamine, cocaine and methylphenidate, rather than antidepressants. Thus, low levels of combined NET plus DAT inhibition may be ideal for a non-abusable antidepressant like bupropion.

Bupropion may be useful in treating nicotine addiction due to its ability to occupy DATs in the striatum and nucleus accumbens, mitigating cravings but not becoming abusable itself. Bupropion was originally marketed in the United States only, and in an immediate-release formulation. Recent formulations have been developed in twice-daily (bupropion SR) and once-daily doses (bupropion XR). These advances not only provide convenience but are also beneficial in reducing the risk of seizures at peak plasma drug levels associated with the original formulation. Bupropion is generally a stimulating agent, and does not appear to cause sexual dysfunction that may be associated with use of other antidepressants. Bupropion has been very useful for patients who experience reduced positive affect, or the "dopamine-deficiency syndrome" (see Fig. 1.35). Oftentimes, augmentation with bupropion to an existing SSRI or SNRI can be useful for patients who have not responded to previous serotonergic-focused treatment.

Bupropion: Tips and Pearls

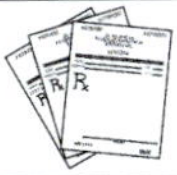

Dosing

Formulation:
Bupropion: 75, 100 mg tablets. SR: 100, 150 and 200 mg tablets. XL: 150 and 300 mg tablets

Dosage Range:
Bupropion: 225-450 mg in 3 divided doses (150 mg maximum single dose). SR: 200-450 mg in 2 divided doses (200 mg maximum single dose). XL: 150-450 mg once/day (450 mg max dose)

Approved For:
Major depressive disorder and nicotine addiction; seasonal affective disorder (XL)

Pearls

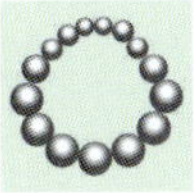

May improve cognitive slowing. Reduces hypersomnia and fatigue. May be effective if SSRIs have failed, or with "poop out"

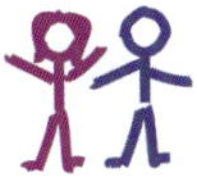

Use with caution in children. Dose may need to be lower initially. May be used for ADHD in children and adolescents and for smoking cessation in adolescents. Watch for induction of mania or suicidal ideation

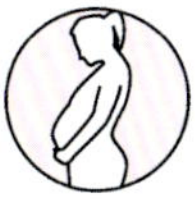

Pregnancy risk category C (some animal studies show adverse effects, no controlled studies in humans)

Side effects I

Weight Gain

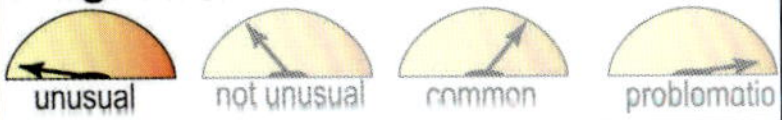

Sedation

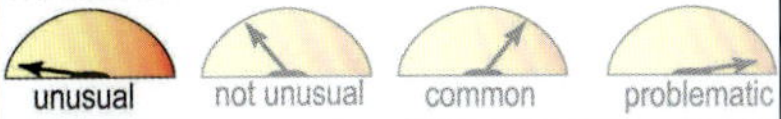

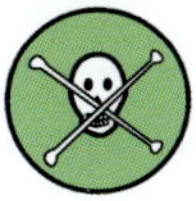

Rare seizures, induction of mania and suicidality

Side effects II

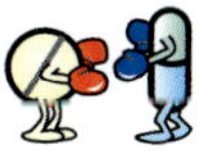

Via weak CYP450 2D6 inhibition, may increase concentrations of other drugs. Do not use with MAOIs, thioridazine

Use with caution in patients with cardiovascular disease

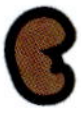

Monitor patients with renal impairment closely. Lower initial dose, give less frequently

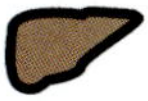

Monitor patients with hepatic impairment closely. Lower initial dose, give less frequently

FIGURE 3.5. Dosing and interaction information for bupropion.

Atomoxetine

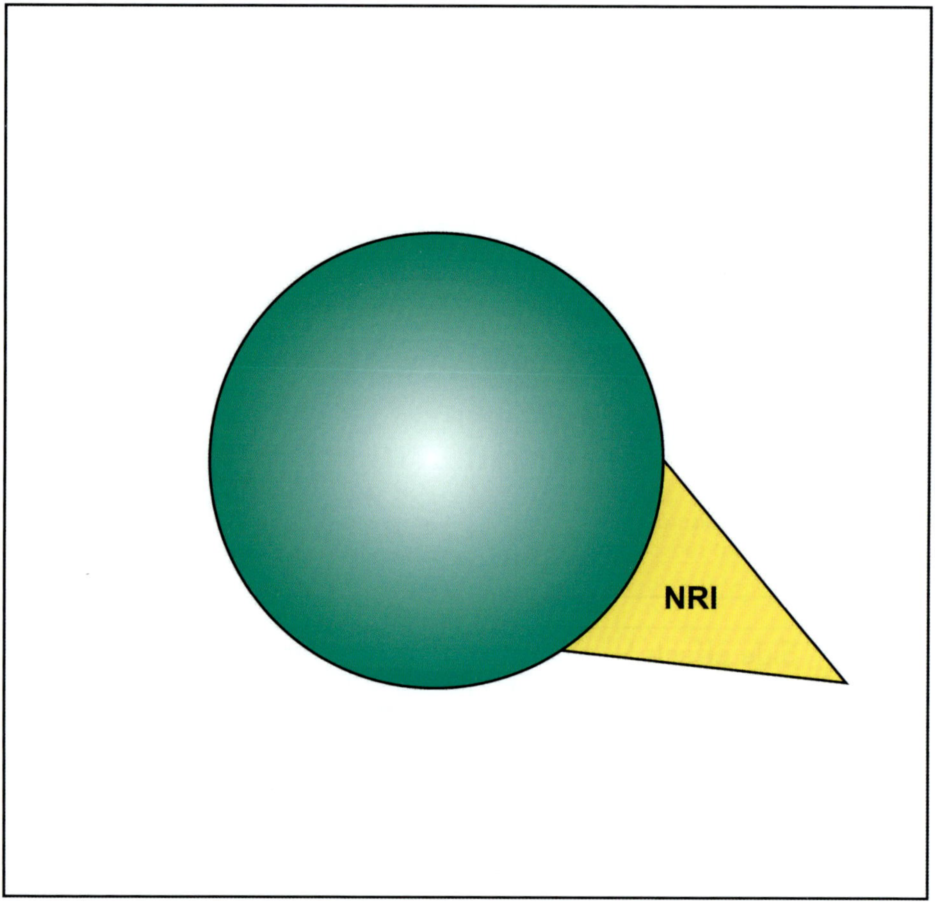

FIGURE 3.6. Atomoxetine was never developed as an antidepressant in the United States, and it is currently marketed only for attention deficit hyperactivity disorder (ADHD). Nevertheless, due to its mechanism of action as an NRI (norepinephrine reuptake inhibitor), it may be useful when given as an augmenting agent with SSRIs or other agents for treatment-resistant depression.

Atomoxetine: Tips and Pearls

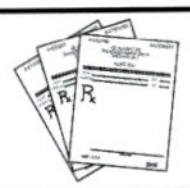

Dosing

Formulation:
10, 18, 25, 40, 60, 80 and 100 mg capsules

Dosage Range:
40-100 mg/day for adults, 0.5-1.2 mg/kg/day for children up to 70 kg

Approved For:
Attention deficit hyperactivity disorder in adults and children over 6

Pearls

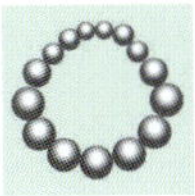

Enhances both DA and NE in prefrontal cortex aiding in attention and concentration. Approved for use in ADHD; does not have abuse potential and is not a scheduled substance

Use with caution in children with depression. Watch for induction of mania or suicidal ideation

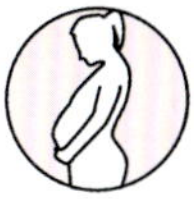

Pregnancy risk category C (some animal studies show adverse effects, no controlled studies in humans)

Side effects I

Weight Gain

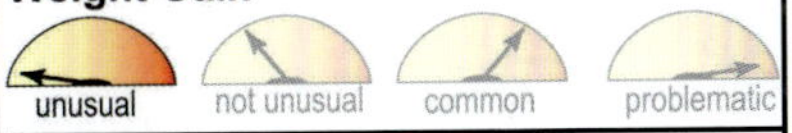

Sedation

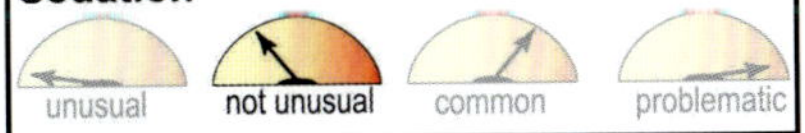

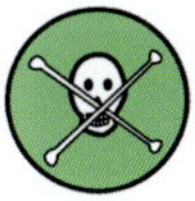

Increased heart rate and hypertension. Rare induction of mania and suicidality. Rare severe liver damage

Side effects II

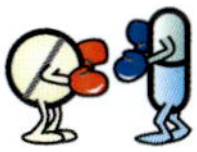

Inhibitors of CYP450 2D6 may increase plasma levels and require dosage reduction of atomoxetine. Co-administration with albuterol may lead to increase in heart rate and blood pressure. Do not use with MAOIs

Use with caution in patients with cardiac impairment; can increase heart rate and blood pressure

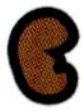

Dose adjustment not generally necessary for renal impairment

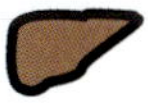

Moderate liver impairment requires 50% of normal dose; severe liver impairment requires 25% of normal dose

FIGURE 3.7. Dosing and interaction information for atomoxetine.

Reboxetine

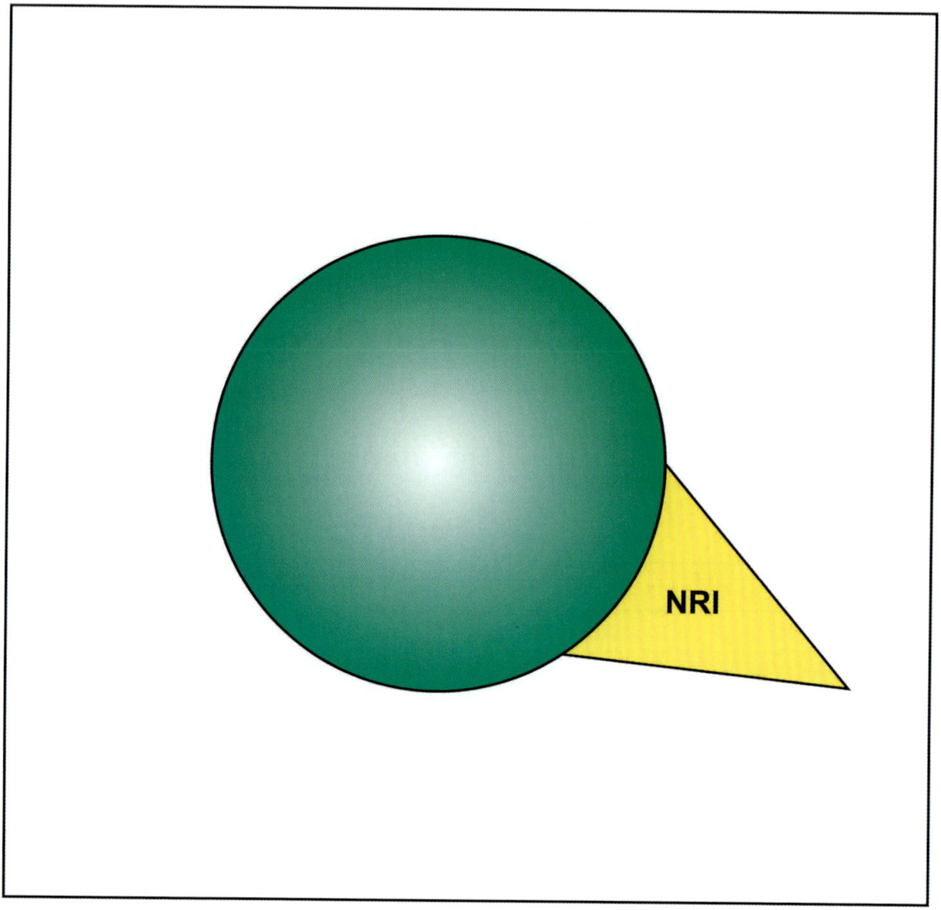

FIGURE 3.8. Reboxetine is approved as an antidepressant in Europe, but not in the United States. Reboxetine may be useful either as a monotherapy or as an augmenting agent in treatment-resistant depression, similar to atomoxetine (see Fig. 3.6), or on its own as a monotherapy after SSRIs have failed or "pooped out."

Reboxetine: Tips and Pearls

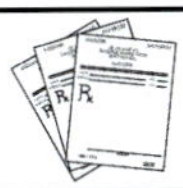

Dosing

Formulation:
2 mg, 4 mg scored tablets

Dosage Range:
8 mg/day in 2 doses (10 mg usual maximum daily dosage)

Approved For:
Commonly prescribed for major depressive disorder, dysthymia, panic disorder and ADHD, though not FDA-approved

Pearls

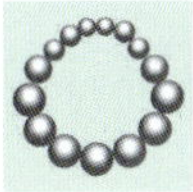

May be more likely than SSRIs to improve social and work functioning. Side effects may appear "anticholinergic," though muscarinic receptors are not blocked directly. Antidotes for the side effects (e.g., constipation, dry mouth, urinary retention) include alpha 1 antagonists such as tamsulosin

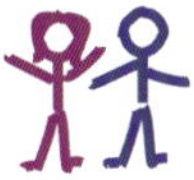

Use with caution in children. Watch for induction of mania or suicidal ideation

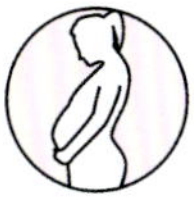

Not generally recommended for use during pregnancy, especially in first trimester

Side effects I

Weight Gain

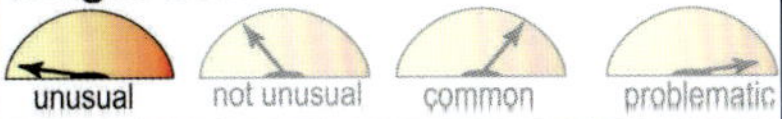

Sedation

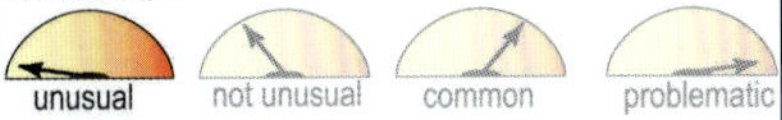

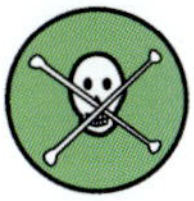

Rare seizures, induction of mania and suicidality

Side effects II

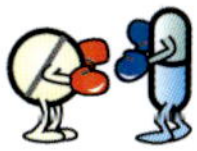

Via CYP450 2D6 and 3A4 inhibition, may increase concentrations of other drugs. Hypokalemia may occur if taken with diuretics. Ergotamine may increase blood pressure. Do not use with MAOIs, thioridazine, pimozide

Use with caution in patients with cardiac impairment

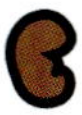

Plasma concentrations increased with renal impairment; may need to lower dose

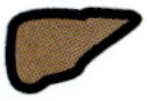

Plasma concentrations increased with hepatic impairment; may need to lower dose

FIGURE 3.9. Dosing and interaction information for reboxetine.

Stahl's Illustrated

Chapter 4

Alpha 2 Antagonists as Serotonin and Norepinephrine Disinhibitors (SNDIs) and Serotonin Antagonist/Reuptake Inhibitors (SARIs)

This chapter reviews the actions of antidepressant drugs that work as alpha 2 antagonists (i.e., mirtazapine) or as serotonin antagonist/reuptake inhibitors (SARIs) (i.e., trazodone and nefazodone). The focus is on the unique characteristics of alpha 2 antagonism and SARIs, both of which are second-line treatment options. The aim is to familiarize the reader with these various options for treating depression.

Symbols Used in this Chapter			
	Life-threatening or Dangerous Side Effects		Drug Interactions
	Tips and Pearls		Cardiac Impairment
	Children and Adolescents		Renal Impairment
	Pregnancy		Hepatic Impairment

Alpha 2 Antagonists and Serotonin Antagonist/Reuptake Inhibitors as Second-Line Treatments

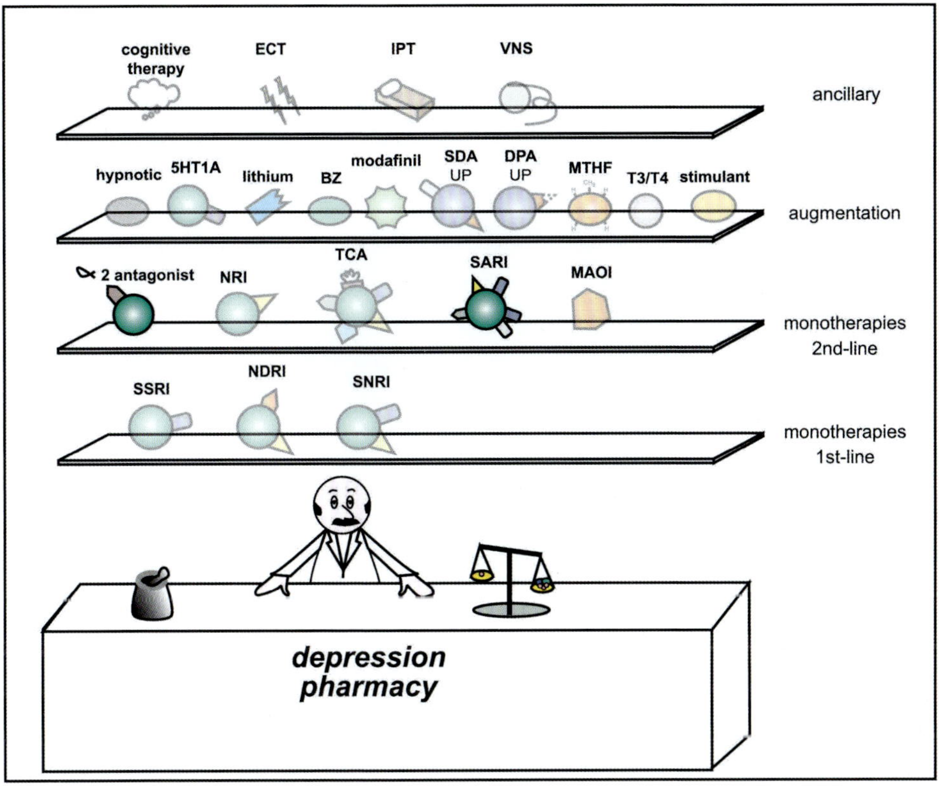

FIGURE 4.1. The alpha 2 antagonist mirtazapine and the SARIs trazodone and nefazodone are listed as second-line monotherapies. They may be useful as monotherapies in situations where patients have not experienced full remission while taking an SSRI and/or SNRI, or as augmentation and/or combination strategies with SSRIs/SNRIs.

SSRI: selective serotonin reuptake inhibitors. NDRI: norepinephrine dopamine reuptake inhibitors. SNRI: serotonin norepinephrine reuptake inhibitors. SDA: serotonin dopamine antagonists. α 2 antagonist: alpha 2 antagonists. NRI: selective norepinephrine reuptake inhibitors. TCA: tricyclic antidepressants. SARI: serotonin 2A antagonist/reuptake inhibitors. MAOI: monoamine oxidase inhibitors. 5HT1A: serotonin 1A partial agonists. BZ: benzodiazepines. DPA: dopamine partial agonists. MTHF: L-5-methyltetrahydrofolate. T3/T4: thyroid hormone. ECT: electroconvulsive therapy. IPT: interpersonal therapy. VNS: vagus nerve stimulation.

Alpha 2 Antagonists (SNDIs or Serotonin Norepinephrine Disinhibitors)

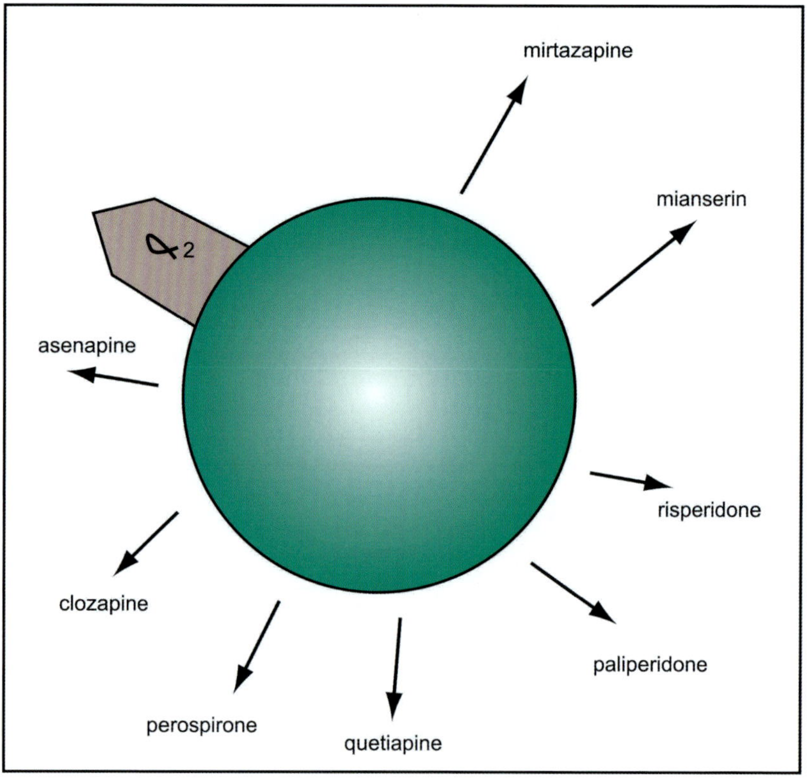

FIGURE 4.2. Unlike SNRIs, alpha 2 antagonists do not block monoamine transporters to achieve their therapeutic effects. Administering an alpha 2 antagonist, which blocks alpha 2 receptors, results in norepinephrine no longer able to turn off its own release. This causes "disinhibition" (i.e., an increase) in norepinephrine release (see Fig. 4.3). Similarly, alpha 2 antagonists do not allow norepinephrine to turn off serotonin release, resulting in "disinhibition" (i.e., an increase in serotonin release; see Fig. 4.4) as well. An additional mechanism of alpha 2 antagonists which aids in increase of serotonin release is the disinhibition of norepinephrine in the noradrenergic pathway to the midbrain raphe (see Figs. 1.25 and 1.26). Norepinephrine neurons from the locus coeruleus innervate cell bodies of serotonergic neurons in the midbrain raphe; thus, this pathway enhances serotonin release via stimulation of alpha 1 receptors with an alpha 2 antagonist. Therefore, alpha 2 antagonists are serotonin and norepinephrine disinhibitors (SNDIs), with dual action increases of both NE and 5HT release.

Alpha 2 Antagonists' Mechanism of Action

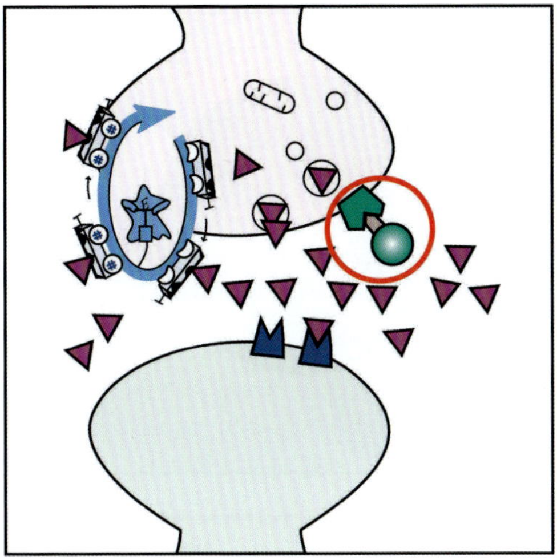

FIGURE 4.3. Alpha 2 antagonists increase noradrenergic neurotransmission via "cutting the brake cable" by blocking presynaptic alpha 2 autoreceptors, causing NE release to become disinhibited, i.e., increased.

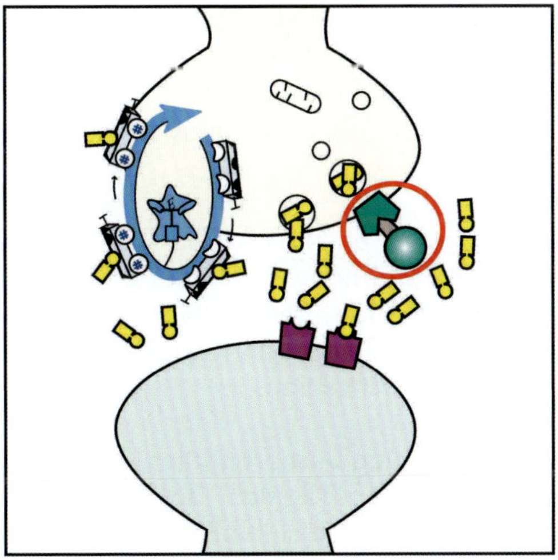

FIGURE 4.4. Additionally, the brake cable is cut for serotonergic neurotransmission via blockade of alpha 2 heteroreceptors, resulting in disinhibition of 5HT release.

Mirtazapine

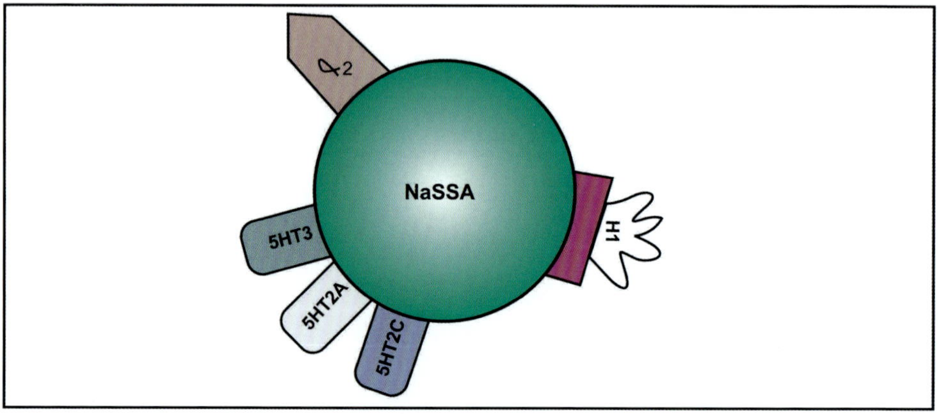

FIGURE 4.5. Mirtazapine has a complex but very interesting pharmacology. It has been called a noradrenergic and specific serotonergic antidepressant (NaSSA), with actions at alpha 2 receptors as well as at three 5HT receptors—2A, 2C and 3. In addition, mirtazapine blocks histamine 1 (H1) receptors. By blocking alpha 2 receptors, mirtazapine increases both serotonin and norepinephrine and is thus a serotonin and norepinephrine disinhibitor or SNDI, as explained in Fig. 4.3. Mirtazapine administration thus causes serotonin to be released onto all receptors; however, since 5HT2A, 5HT2C and 5HT3 receptors are blocked by mirtazapine, the net stimulation falls on the 5HT1A receptors. This further results in release of dopamine (see Figs. 1.32 and 1.33), which may be helpful in depression as well as anxiety.

Mirtazapine's antagonist actions at 5HT2A and 2C receptors also results in increased release of dopamine and norepinephrine, and these 5HT2A and 5HT2C antagonist actions may also provide useful anxiolytic and antidepressant as well as sleep-restoring properties. In addition, mirtazapine is able to increase serotonin release without causing sexual dysfunction.

Due to its 5HT2A and 5HT2C antagonist properties, and thus its ability to disinhibit both NE and DA release (see Figs. 1.32 and 1.33), mirtazapine is further classified as a norepinephrine and dopamine disinhibitor (NDDI). 5HT3 antagonist action may reduce nausea, with H1 action potentially relieving insomnia and improving anxiety, but causing weight gain. So, this complex molecule is an NDDI (due to 5HT2A and 5HT2C antagonism), an SNDI (due to alpha 2 antagonism) plus a 5HT3 and H1 antagonist!

Mirtazapine: Tips and Pearls

Dosing

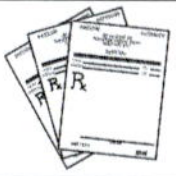

Formulation:
15 and 30 mg scored, 45 mg tablets. SolTab disintegrating tablets 15, 30 and 45 mg

Dosage Range:
15-45 mg at night

Approved For:
Major depressive disorder

Pearls

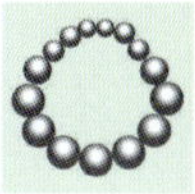

Rarely causes sexual dysfunction. Does not interfere with CYP450 system. Adding alpha 2 antagonism to 5HT and/or NE reuptake blockers such as SSRIs or SNRIs may be synergistic for severe depression

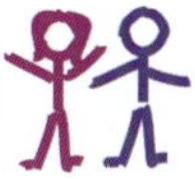

Use with caution in children. Watch for induction of mania or suicidal ideation

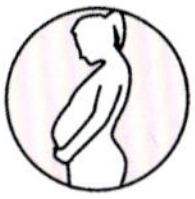

Pregnancy risk category C (some animal studies show adverse effects, no controlled studies in humans)

Side effects I

Weight Gain

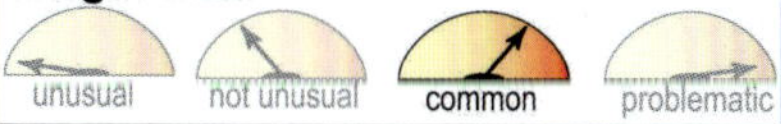

Sedation

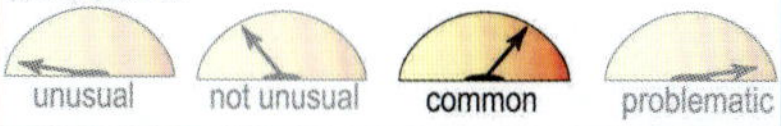

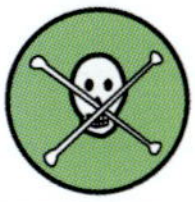

Rare seizures, induction of mania and suicidality

Side effects II

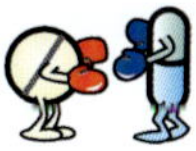

No significant pharmacokinetic drug interactions. Do not use with MAOIs

Use with caution in patients with cardiovascular disease

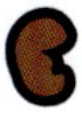

Use with caution in patients with renal problems

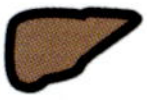

Use with caution in patients with hepatic complications

FIGURE 4.6. Dosing and interaction information for mirtazapine.

Serotonin Antagonist/Reuptake Inhibitors (SARIs)

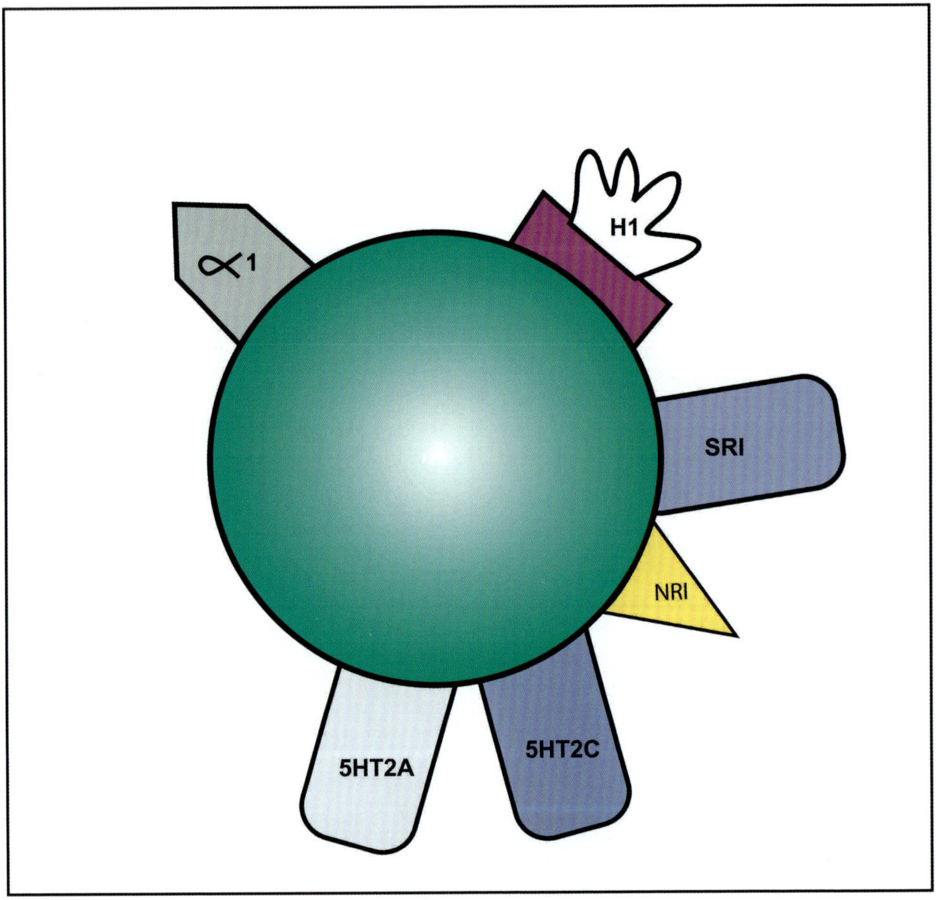

FIGURE 4.7. Serotonin 2A antagonist/reuptake inhibitors (SARIs) block 5HT2A and 5HT2C receptors, the 5HT transporter (SRI) and alpha 1 adrenergic receptors. Trazodone also has histamine 1 receptor antagonism properties, whereas nefazodone also blocks the NE transporter (NRI).

Mechanism of Action of SARIs: Parts 1-4

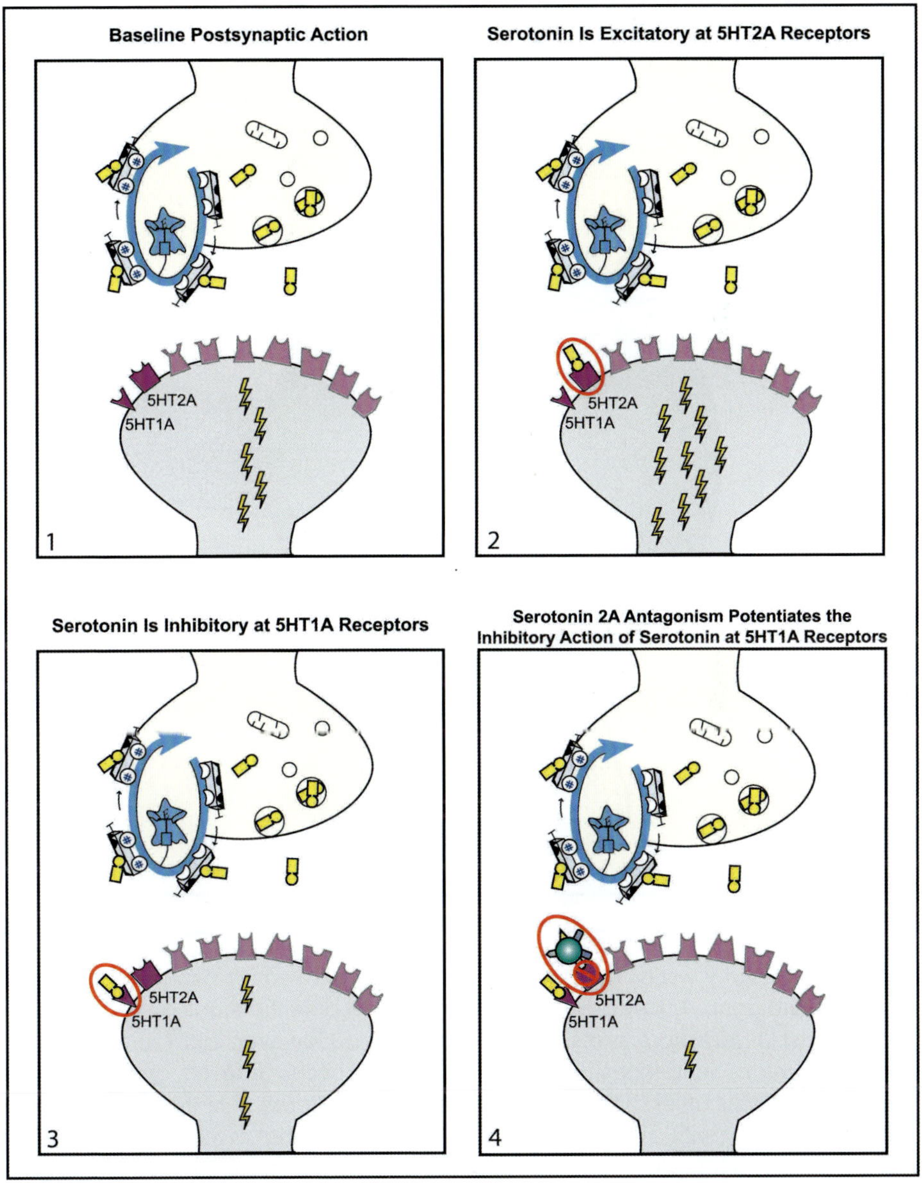

FIGURE 4.8.

Trazodone

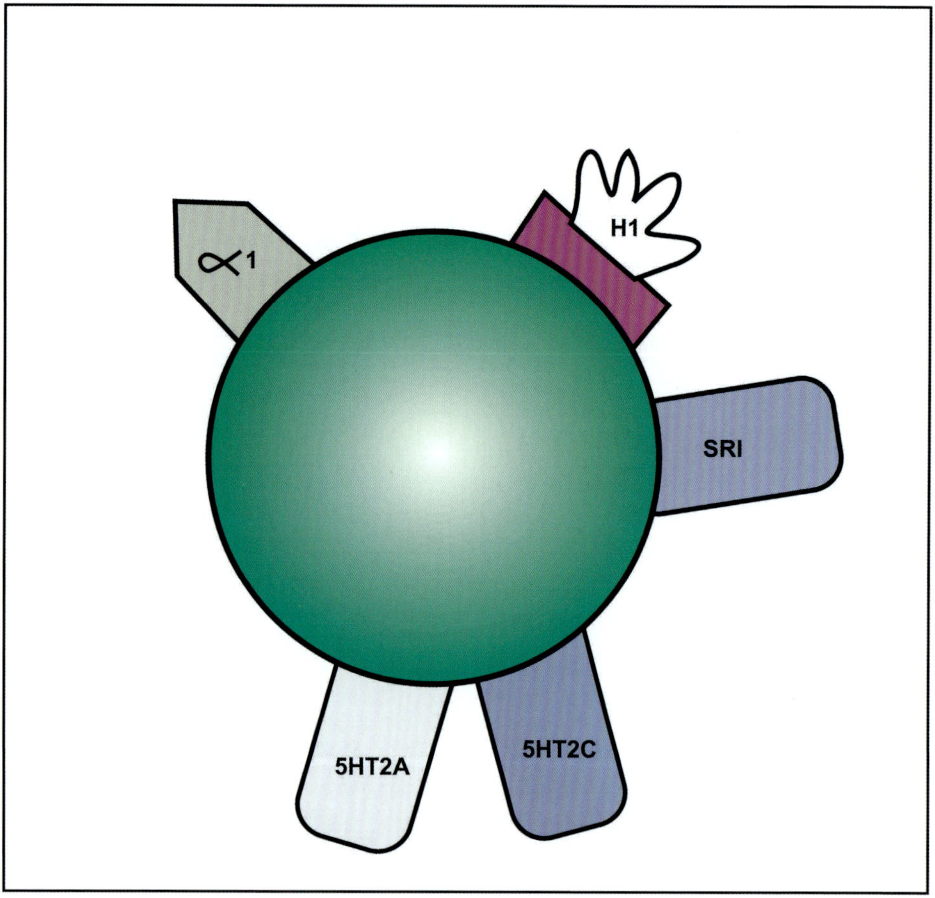

FIGURE 4.9. In many ways, trazodone is two drugs: a low-dose hypnotic and a high-dose antidepressant. At low doses, trazodone's most potent actions at 5HT2A, alpha 1 and even H1 receptors provide hypnotic action. However, SERT blockade from serotonin reuptake inhibition (SRI actions) does not occur at levels great enough to increase 5HT levels unless trazodone is given in high doses. It is this SERT blockade working in synergy with 5HT2A and 5HT2C antagonism that gives trazodone its ability to act as an antidepressant (see Fig. 4.8) and why it is called a SARI (serotonin 2A/2C antagonist and reuptake inhibitor) at high doses. Trazodone lacks sexual side effects because of this SARI action.

Trazodone: Tips and Pearls

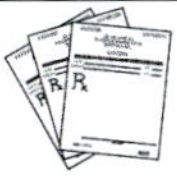

Dosing

Formulation:
50 and 100 mg scored, 150 mg tablets, 150 and 300 mg with pividone scored

Dosage Range:
150-600 mg/day

Approved For:
Depression

Pearls

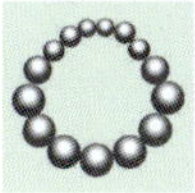

Rarely causes sexual dysfunction. Expert psychopharmacologists may utilize trazodone for insomnia associated with MAOI use. Patient must be closely monitored

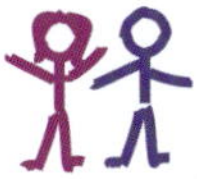

Children require lower initial dose and slow titration. Boys may be more sensitive to prolonged erections than adult men. Use with caution in children. Watch for induction of mania or suicidal ideation

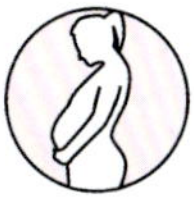

Pregnancy risk category C (some animal studies show adverse effects, no controlled studies in humans)

Side effects I

Weight Gain

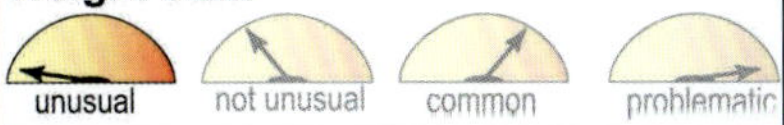

Sedation

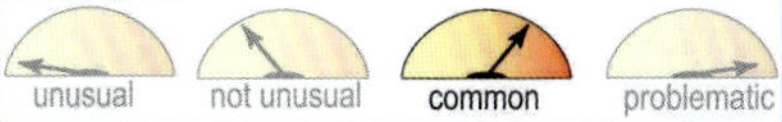

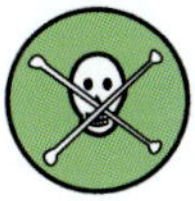

Rare priapism, seizures, induction of mania and suicidality

Side effects II

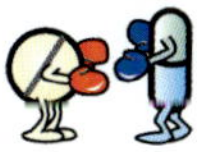

Some SSRIs may raise plasma trazodone levels. Prothrombin time may be affected in patients taking trazodone and warfarin. May block hypotensive effects of some antihypertensive drugs. Do not use with MAOIs (see Pearls)

May be arrhythmogenic; monitor patients with cardiac impairment closely

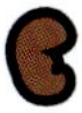

No dose adjustment necessary for renal impairment

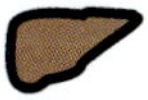

Use with caution in patients with hepatic impairments

FIGURE 4.10. Dosing and interaction information for trazodone.

Nefazodone

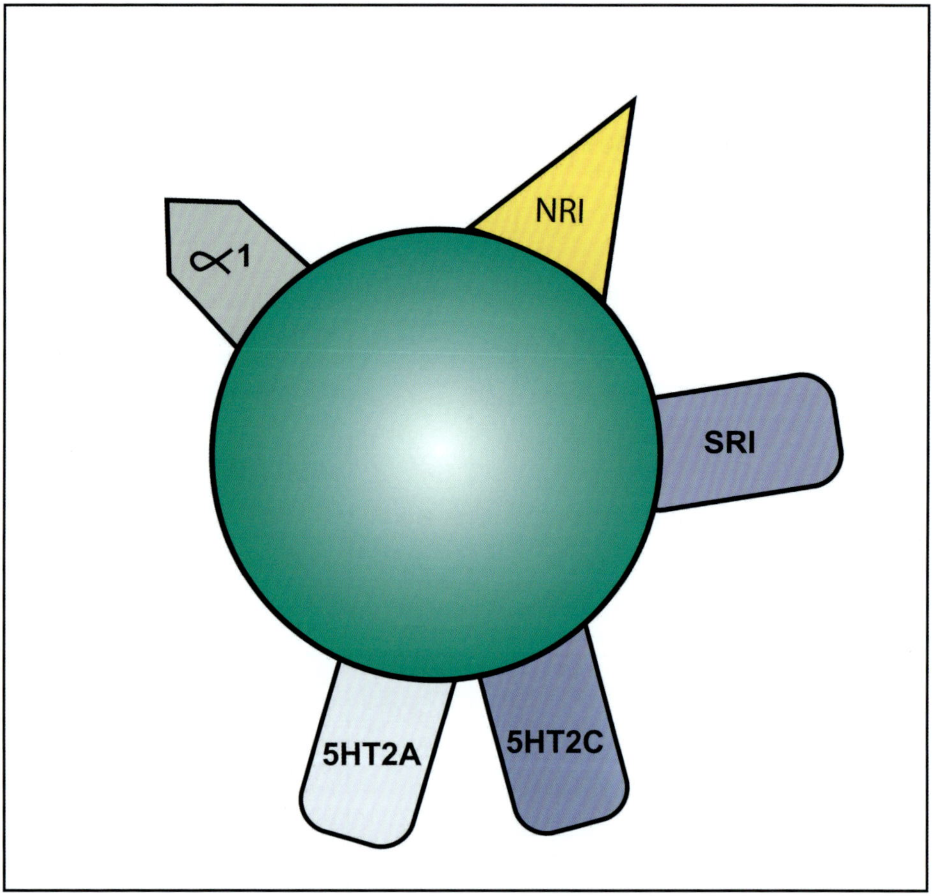

FIGURE 4.11. Nefazodone has strong 5HT2A antagonist actions with weaker 5HT2C antagonism and weaker SERT inhibition. This particular drug is currently not used very often due to the potential for rare liver toxicity.

Nefazodone: Tips and Pearls

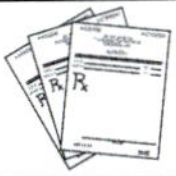

Dosing

Formulation:
50, 200 and 250 mg tablets, 100 and 150 mg scored

Dosage Range:
300-600 mg/day

Approved For:
Depression, relapse prevention in major depressive disorder

Pearls

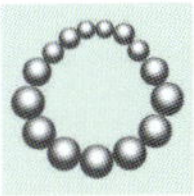

Cognitive behavioral therapy can enhance efficacy of nefazodone in depression. Risk of hepatotoxicity makes nefazodone second-line choice; has been pulled from some markets

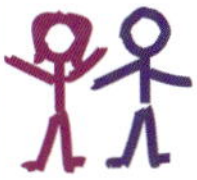

Use with caution, if at all, in children. Watch for induction of mania or suicidal ideation

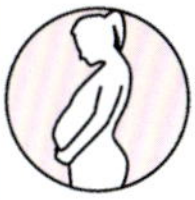

Pregnancy risk category C (some animal studies show adverse effects, no controlled studies in humans)

Side effects I

Weight Gain

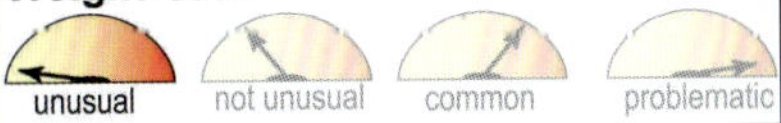

Sedation

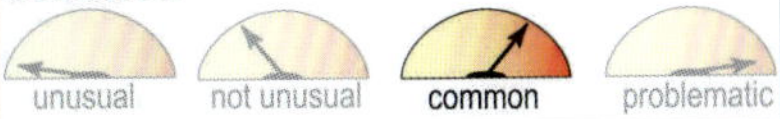

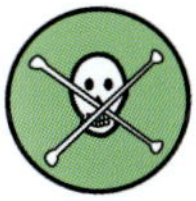

Rare seizures, induction of mania, suicidality and priapism. Hepatic failure requiring liver transplant and/or fatal

Side effects II

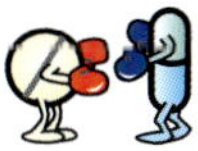

mCPP, metabolite of nefazodone, is substrate of CYP450 2D6; combination with 2D6 inhibitors will raise levels leading to 5HT2C receptor stimulation and dizziness/agitation. Via CYP450 3A4 inhibition, concentrations of other drugs may be increased. Do not use with MAOIs, pimozide, carbamazepine

Use with caution in patients with cardiovascular issues

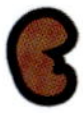

No dose adjustment necessary for renal impairment

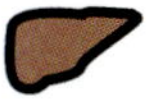

Contraindicated in patients with known hepatic impairment. Rare liver failure, hepatic transplants and death

FIGURE 4.12. Dosing and interaction information for nefazodone.

Stahl's Illustrated | Chapter 5

Monoamine Oxidase Inhibitors (MAOIs) and Tricyclic Antidepressants (TCAs)

This chapter reviews the classical antidepressants known as monoamine oxidase inhibitors (MAOIs) and tricyclic antidepressants (TCAs). The focus here is on mechanisms of action of these particular classes. The aim of this chapter is to familiarize the reader with these "old-fashioned" but quite powerful options for treating depression.

MAOIs and TCAs as Second-Line Treatments

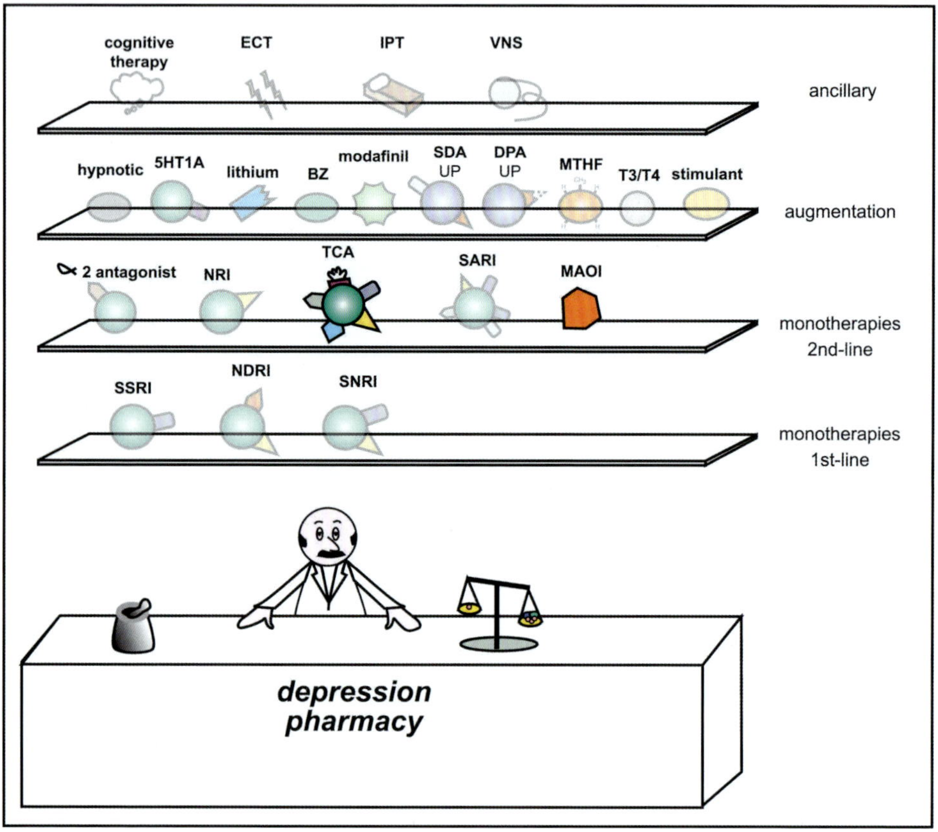

FIGURE 5.1. MAOIs and TCAs are generally considered second- or third-line monotherapies. These agents may be utilized in difficult-to-treat cases, where other first-line treatments may have failed to produce results.

SSRI: selective serotonin reuptake inhibitors. NDRI: norepinephrine dopamine reuptake inhibitors. SNRI: serotonin norepinephrine reuptake inhibitors. SDA: serotonin dopamine antagonists. α 2 antagonist: alpha 2 antagonists. NRI: selective norepinephrine reuptake inhibitors. TCA: tricyclic antidepressants. SARI: serotonin 2A antagonist/reuptake inhibitors. MAOI: monoamine oxidase inhibitors. 5HT1A: serotonin 1A partial agonists. BZ: benzodiazepines. DPA: dopamine partial agonists. MTHF: L-5-methyl-tetrahydrofolate. T3/T4: thyroid hormone. ECT: electroconvulsive therapy. IPT: interpersonal therapy. VNS: vagus nerve stimulation.

Properties of Tricyclic Antidepressants

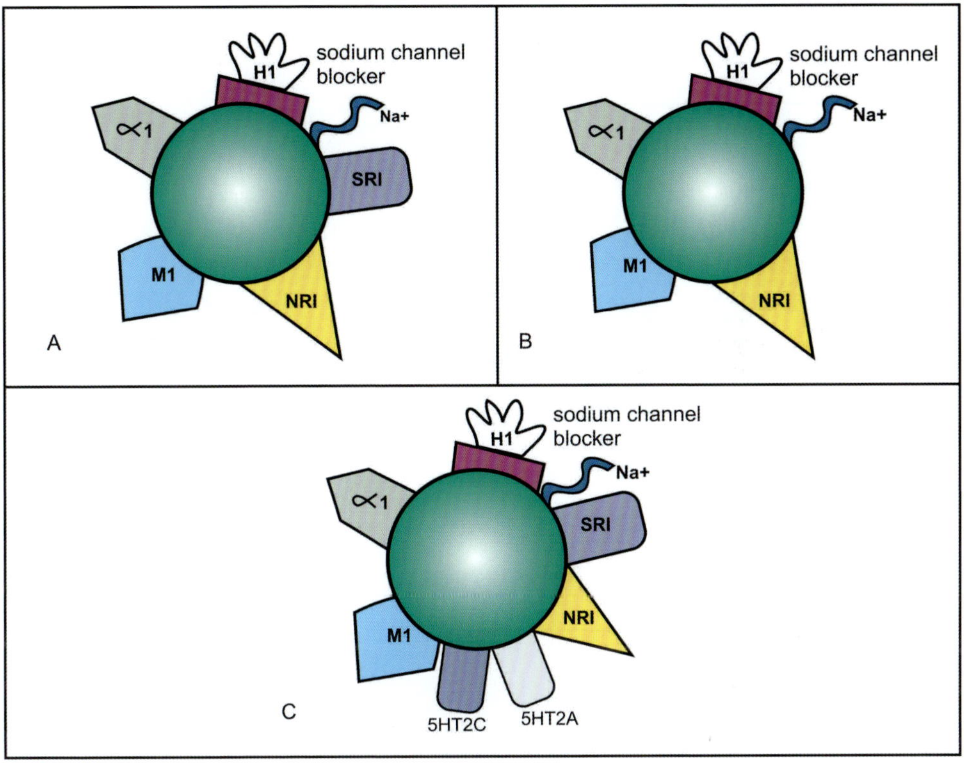

FIGURE 5.2. All tricyclics block NET (the norepinephrine transporter; they are NRIs, or norepinephrine reuptake inhibitors); some block SERT (the serotonin transporter; they are SRIs, or serotonin reuptake inhibitors) as well, both properties which can lead to an antidepressant effect (A). In addition, all TCAs share the secondary properties of inhibition of histamine 1, alpha 1 and muscarinic cholinergic receptors (M1) (B), and some have additional antagonist properties at 5HT2C and 5HT2A receptors (C). Tricyclics block voltage-sensitive sodium channels, which is why they can be lethal in overdose (see Fig. 5.6).

Therapeutic Actions of Tricyclic Antidepressants: Part 1

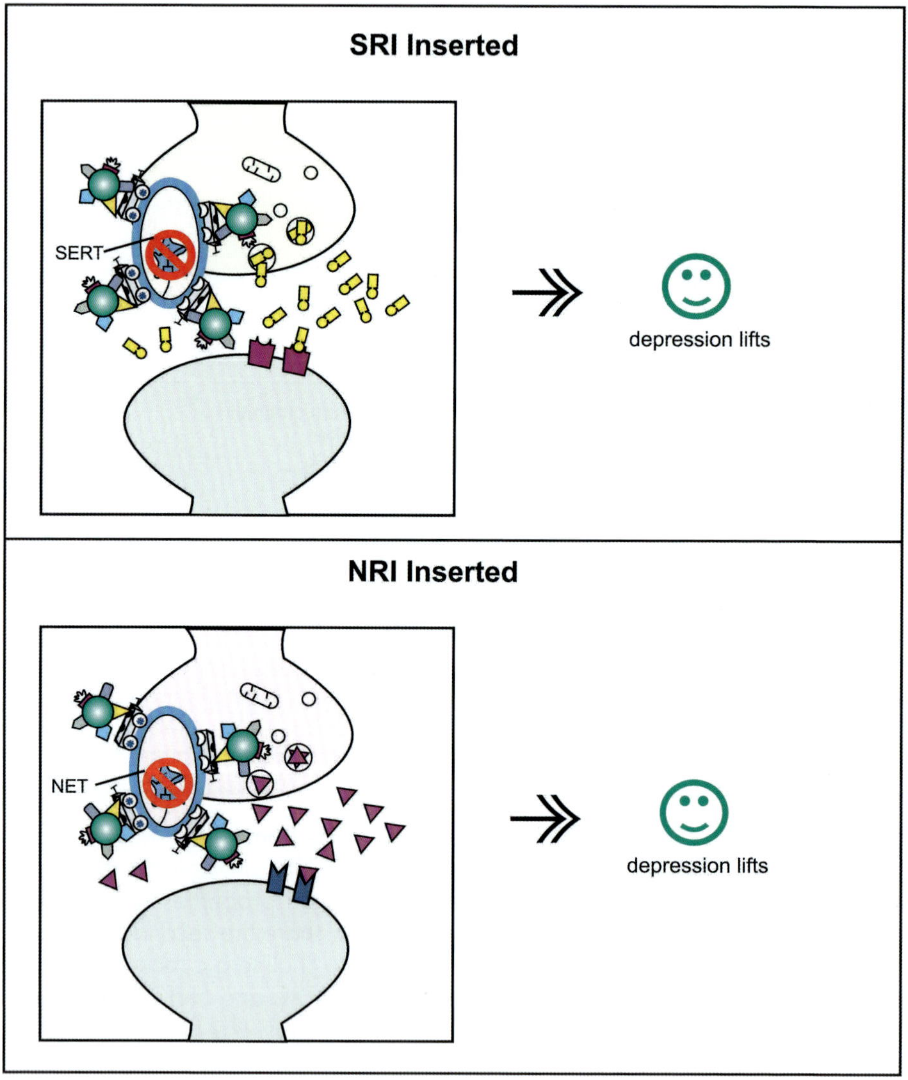

FIGURE 5.3. Here a TCA is depicted inserted into the 5HT reuptake pump, blocking it and causing 5HT accumulation in the synapse and an antidepressant effect (A). Also depicted here is the NRI portion of the TCA inserted to cause synaptic accumulation of NE and an antidepressant effect (B).

Therapeutic Actions of Tricyclic Antidepressants: Part 2

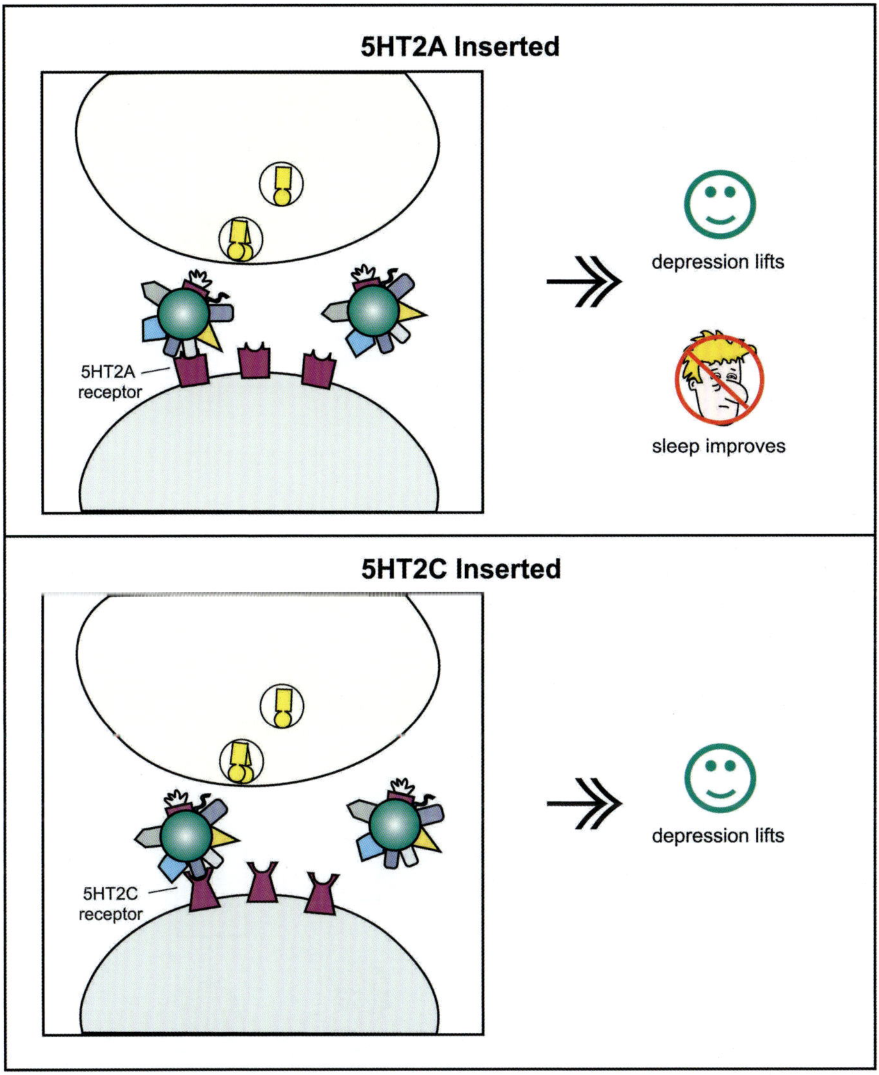

FIGURE 5.4. When TCAs block 5HT2A receptors (A), an antidepressant effect is achieved (perhaps through disinhibition of DA and NE release, as previously discussed). In addition, sleep problems may improve (A). TCAs inserted into the 5HT2C receptors results in their blockade and also produces an antidepressant effect (B), perhaps through disinhibition of DA and NE release as well.

Side Effects of TCAs: Part 1

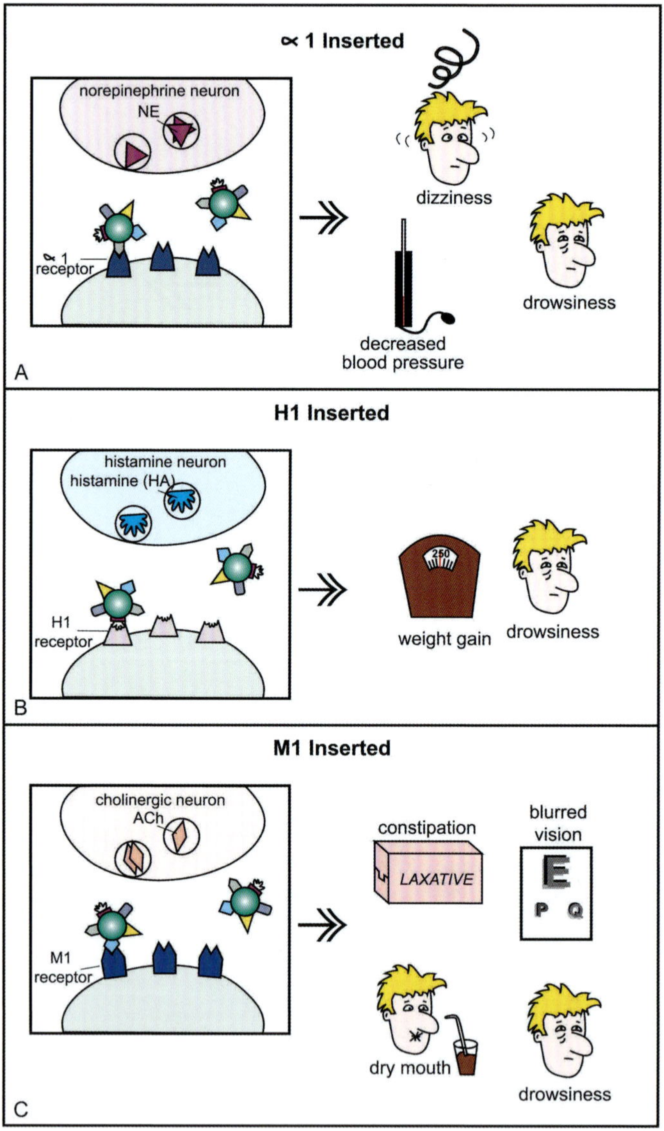

FIGURE 5.5 When TCAs are inserted at each of the receptors indicated above, side effects may ensue. Refer to each part of figure (A, B, C) for respective side effects of TCA receptor binding.

Side Effects of TCAs: Part 2

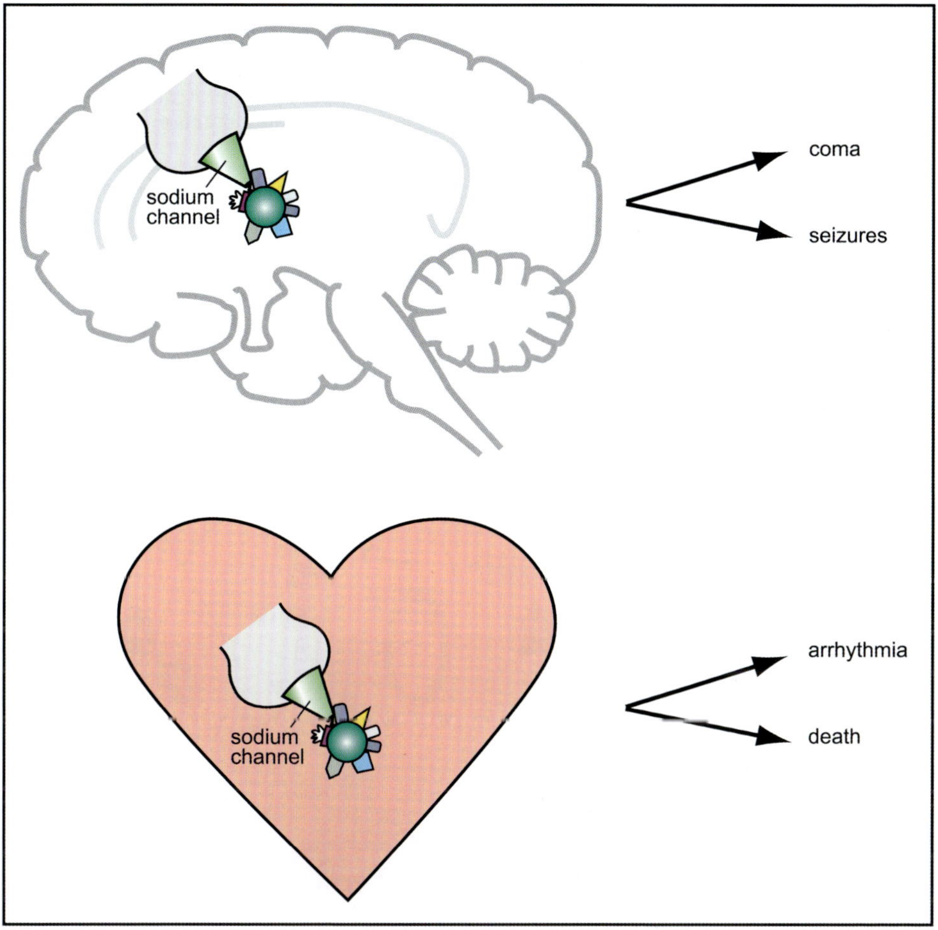

FIGURE 5.6. One of the properties of all TCAs is their ability to block voltage-sensitive sodium channels. When these channels are blocked in the brain and heart, as depicted above, side effects can include coma and seizure (due to central nervous system actions), arrythmia, and death (due to peripheral cardiac actions), especially in overdose.

MAO-A and MAO-B Inhibition and Antidepressant Action

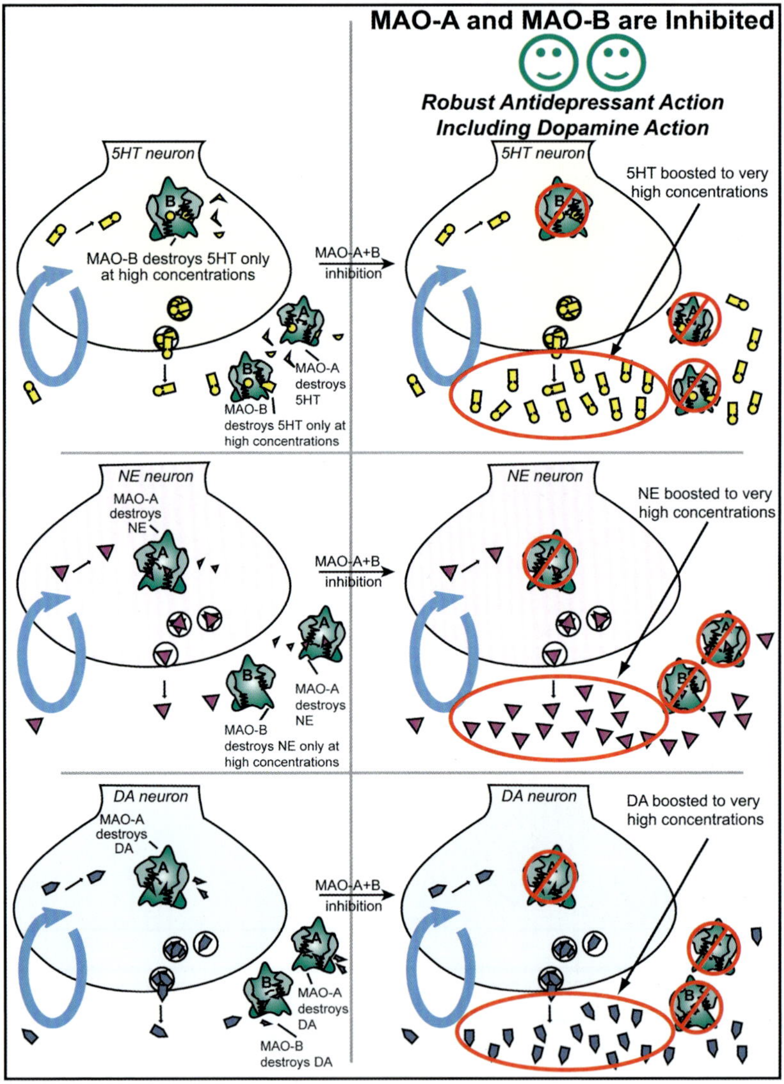

FIGURE 5.7. MAO-A metabolizes serotonin, norepinephrine and dopamine, whereas MAO-B preferentially metabolizes dopamine (left panels). Combined inhibition of MAO-A and MAO-B results in greater increases in all three neurotransmitters compared to does inhibition of just MAO-A or MAO-B (right panels).

MAO Interaction with SRIs

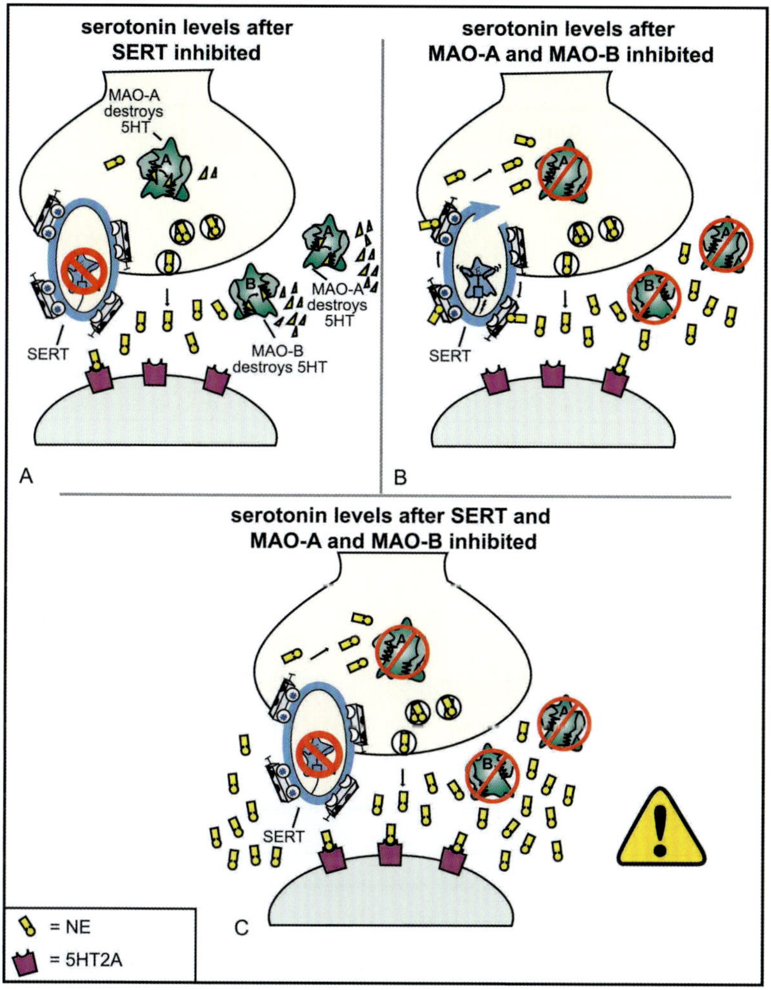

FIGURE 5.8. 5HT is increased by either SERT inhibition by an agent that can block serotonin reuptake, like SSRIs or SNRIs (A) or by MAO inhibition by an MAOI (B). However, when both SERT and MAO are inhibited, 5HT levels can dramatically increase. Thus, excessive stimulation of postsynaptic 5HT receptors can occur to dangerous levels (C) and cause hyperthermia, coma, seizures, cardiovascular problems, and death. This is known as the "serotonin syndrome" and is why the combination of an MAOI with any drug that has SRI properties is strictly contraindicated.

Drugs to Avoid with MAOIs

Drugs With Adrenergic Stimulation			
Decongestants	**Stimulants**	**Antidepressants with NRI**	**Other**
Phenylephrine	Amphetamine	Most tricyclics	Phentermine
Pseudoephedrine	Methylphenidate	NRIs	Local anesthetics containing vasoconstrictors
		SNRIs	Tapentadol
		NDRIs	Cocaine, methamphetamine

A

Drugs With Serotonin Reuptake Inhibition			
Antidepressants	**Drugs of Abuse**	**Opioids**	**Other**
SSRIs	MDMA (ecstasy)	meperidine	non-subcutaneous sumatriptan
SNRIs	cocaine	tramadol	chlorpheniramine
clomipramine	methamphetamine	methadone	brompheniramine
St. John's wort	high-dose or injected amphetamine	fentanyl	dextromethorphan procarbazine?

B

TABLE 5.1 Pharmacotherapeutic agents that, when combined with MAOIs, may result in potentially dangerous hypertensive reactions (A) or potentially lethal combinations causing hyperthermia (B).

Identifying a Hypertensive Crisis and Ways to Avoid It

Hypertensive Crisis

• Defined as having a diastolic blood pressure >120 mmHg
• Potentially fatal reaction characterized by:
  • Occipital headache which may radiate frontally
  • Palpitation
  • Neck stiffness or soreness
  • Nausea
  • Vomiting
  • Sweating (sometimes with fever)
  • Dilated pupils, photophobia
  • Tachycardia or bradycardia that can be associated with constricting chest pain

A

Foods to avoid*	**Foods allowed**
Dried, aged, smoked, fermented, spoiled, or improperly stored meat, poultry, and fish	Fresh or processed meat, poultry, and fish; properly stored pickled or smoked fish
Broad bean pods	All other vegetables
Aged cheeses	Processed cheese slices, cottage cheese, ricotta cheese, yogurt, cream cheese
Tap and unpasteurized beer	Canned or bottled beer and alcohol
Marmite	Brewer's and baker's yeast
Sauerkraut, kimchee	
Soy products/tofu	Peanuts
Banana peel	Bananas, avocados, raspberries
Tyramine-containing nutritional supplement	
	B

TABLE 5.2. Signs of a hypertensive crisis (A), and ways that this crisis may be avoided when using MAOIs (B) with dietary restrictions.

Tyramine Content

Cheese		mg per 15 g serving
English STILTON	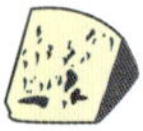	17.3
Kraft ® grated PARMESAN	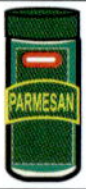	0.2
Philadelphia ® CREAM CHEESE	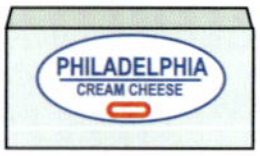	0
Serving		**mg per serving**
1/2 medium double cheese, double pepperoni		0.378
1/2 medium double cheese, double pepperoni		0.063
1/2 medium double cheese, double pepperoni		0
Wine		**mg per 4 oz serving**
Ruffino CHIANTI		0.36
Blue Nun ® WHITE	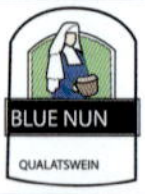	0.32
Cinzano VERMOUTH		0

FIGURE 5.9. Tyramine content for cheeses, pizza and wine. Aged cheeses generally contain the highest concentrations of tyramine, whereas processed cheese, cheese topping on pizza and wine are not as high in tyramine content. For comparisons, "high tyramine meals" are those with 40 mg of tyramine.

Tyramine and Reversible MAOIs

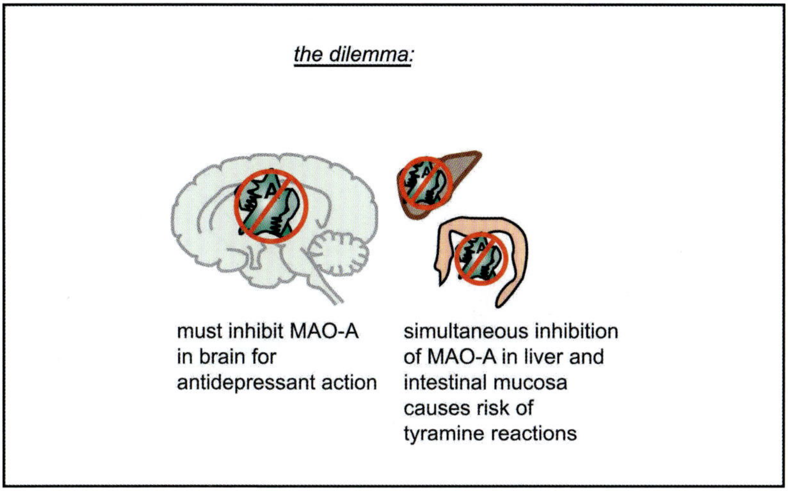

FIGURE 5.10. MAO-A is present in both the brain and gut. Its inhibition in the gut can lead to increased risk of tyramine reaction.

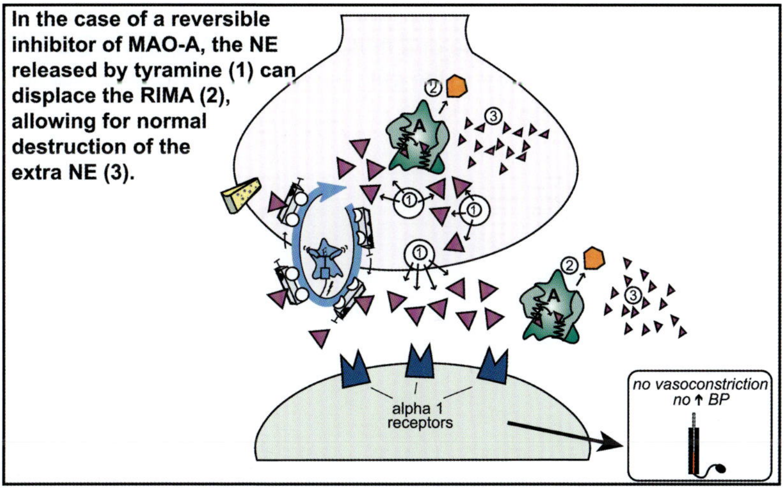

FIGURE 5.11. Reversible MAOs (RIMAs) have a form of enzyme inhibition that can reverse their original action in the presence of increased levels of NE released by tyramine, and thereby remove excess NE from the gut.

Selegiline: Reducing Tyramine Reactions

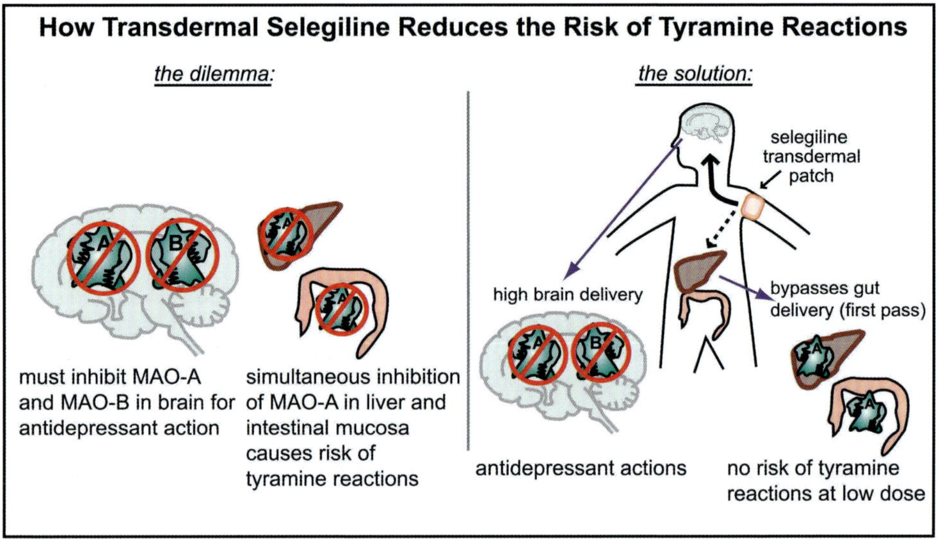

FIGURE 5.12. Transdermal selegiline is one solution for MAO-A and MAO-B antidepressant effects without tyramine reactions. Bypassing the liver via transdermal administration allows for a high dose and thus both MAO-A and MAO-B inhibition in the brain while bypassing delivery to the gut, thus avoiding tyramine reactions due to low MAO-A inhibition in the gut.

Stahl's Illustrated

Chapter 6

Building a Treatment Plan with Novel Treatment and Augmentation Options for Depression

Several emerging treatment options for depression have shown promise, especially for patients resistant to treatment with first-line drugs. Described in this chapter are a variety of options that may assist in treating depression, whether as a monotherapy or in combination with another drug of choice. The concept of trimonoamine modulators (TMMs) is introduced to explain the actions of many agents used to augment antidepressants including lithium, thyroid, and L-methylfolate. Estrogen as a TMM is explained in the following chapter. Various forms of brain stimulation/neuromodulation are also illustrated here, from vagus nerve stimulation (VNS) to transcranial magnetic stimulation (TMS) to deep brain stimulation (DBS). A few new therapeutic approaches to the treatment of depression are also included at the end of the chapter.

Vilazodone

Vilazodone

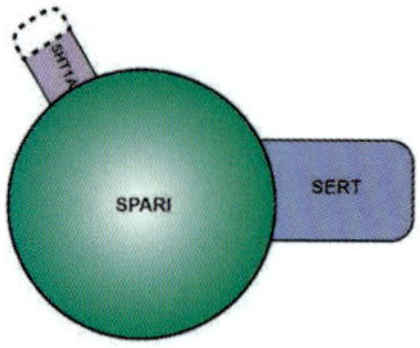

Dosage Range:

40 mg/day

Approved For:

Major depressive disorder

Pearls:

Vilazodone's relative lack of sexual dysfunction and weight gain compared to many other antidepressants that block serotonin reuptake may be due to its serotonin 1A partial agonist properties; high doses would theoretically raise brain serotonin levels more robustly than the standard dose and may improve efficacy in some patients but reduce tolerability in others; consider doses of 50–80 mg daily for patients with treatment-resistant depression or treatment-resistant OCD and other anxiety disorders; consider for patients with comorbid anxiety disorders plus depression; nonresponse to vilazodone in elderly patients may require consideration of mild cognitive impairment or Alzheimer disease; safety and efficacy have not been established in children; Pregnancy Risk Category C; do not use with MAOIs or for at least 21 days after MAOIs are stopped; do not start an MAOI for at least 5 half-lives (5 to 7 days for most drugs) after discontinuing vilazodone; dose should be reduced to 20 mg when co-administered with strong CYP3A4 inhibitors.

TABLE 6.1. Vilazodone was approved to treat major depressive disorder in 2011. It is the first member of a new antidepressant class: serotonin partial agonist reuptake inhibitors, or SPARIs.

Lithium

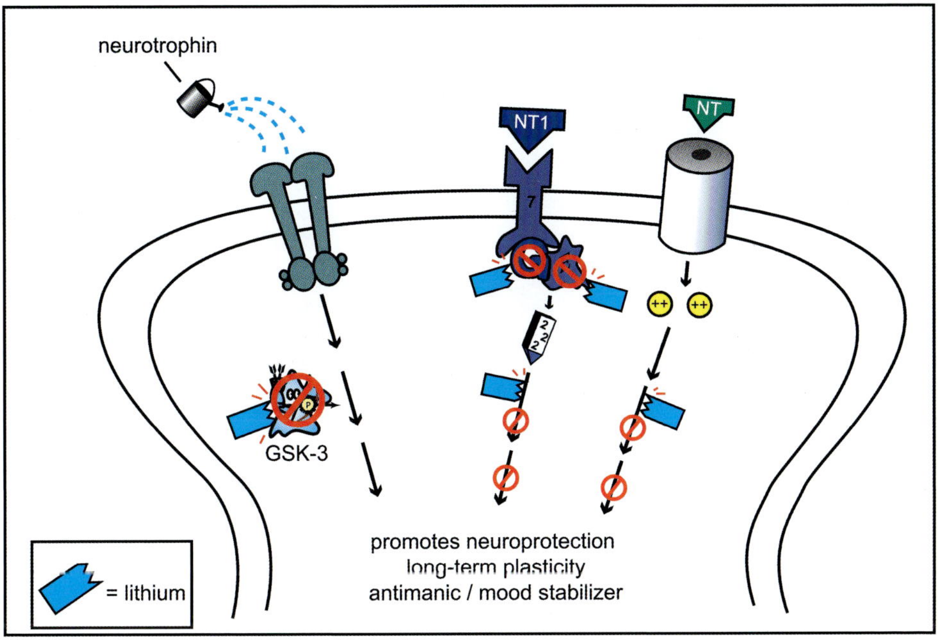

FIGURE 6.1. Although the mechanism of action of lithium is still not completely known, it is posited to act by modulating G proteins (middle), or to inhibit second messenger enzymes such as inositol monophosphate (right), both of which affect signal transduction. Lithium might also act within various downstream signal transduction cascades (left). Lithium can be a useful booster of antidepressant action, both in patients with unipolar depression that is non-responsive to antidepressant monotherapy, and in bipolar depression to augment other mood stabilizers.

Lithium as a Trimonoamine Modulator

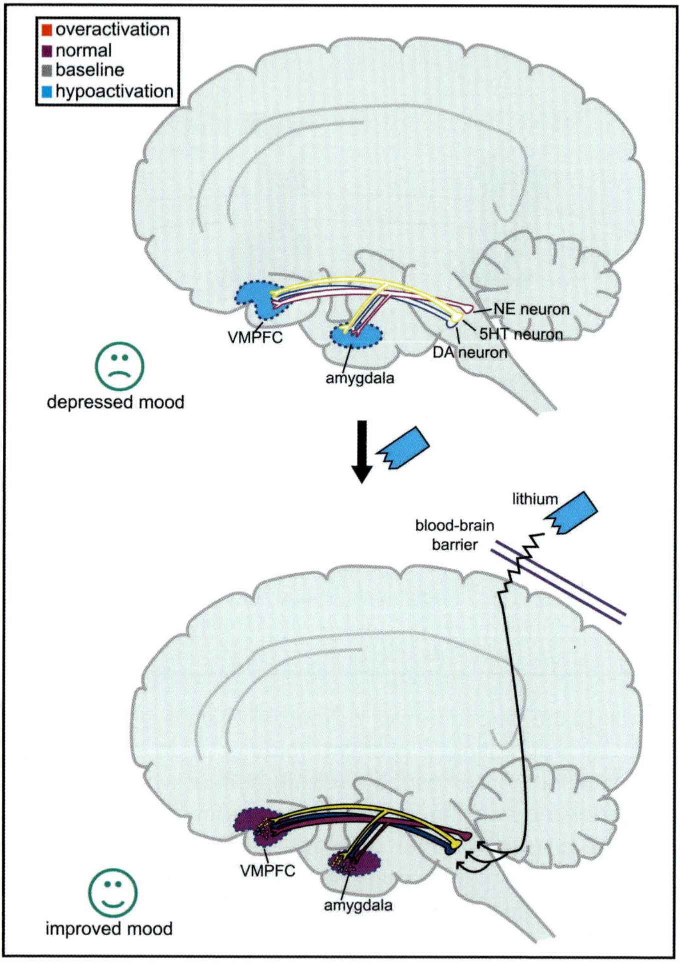

FIGURE 6.2. Lithium can boost the actions of monoamines, purportedly via one of the mechanisms depicted in the previous figure. While the mechanism of action of lithium is still not completely understood, lithium is commonly used as an augmenting agent for patients who have not responded to previous antidepressant treatment. Patients who are theoretically deficient in one or more of the three monoamines (trimonoamines are dopamine, norepinephrine and serotonin; see Fig. 1.9B), despite treatment with an antidepressant (top), can have their monoamine activity theoretically restored when lithium is added (bottom).

Thyroid as a Trimonoamine Modulator

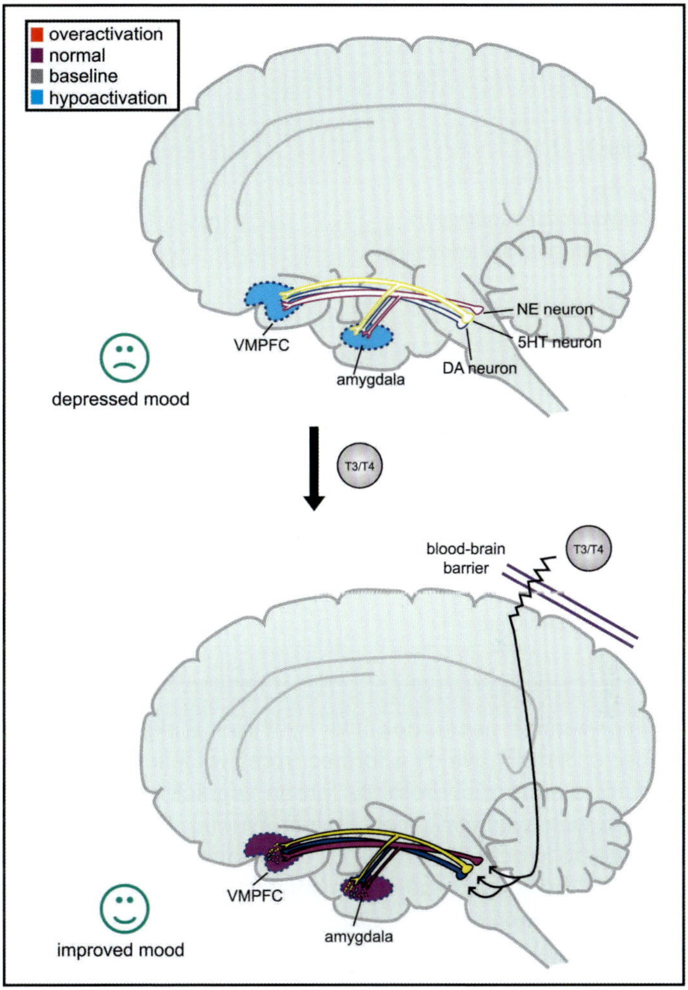

FIGURE 6.3. Thyroid hormone binds to a nuclear hormone receptor that may lead to changes in neuronal gene expression that modulates one or more of the three monoamine neurotransmitters. Thus, thyroid hormone (T3, T4) can be considered a potential trimonoamine modulator (TMM). Patients who are theoretically deficient in one ore more of the three monoamines dopamine, norepinephrine or serotonin (top; see Figs. 1.9B and 6.2), despite treatment with an antidepressant, can have their monoamine activity theoretically restored when thyroid is added (bottom).

How Does L-methylfolate Work? Part 1: L-methylfolate is the Centrally Active Form of the Vitamin Folic Acid

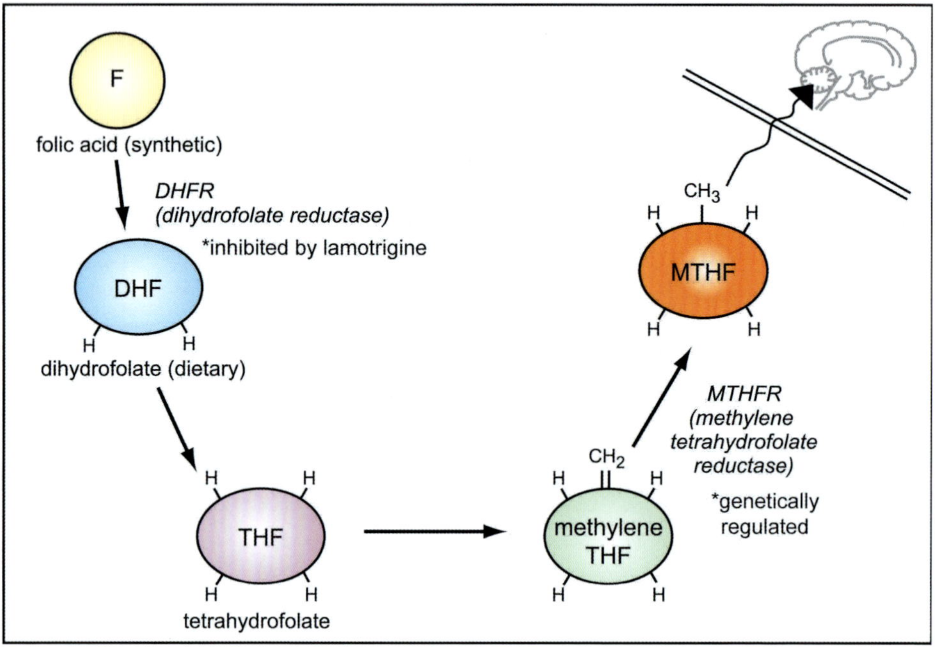

FIGURE 6.4. Trimonoamine neurotransmitter synthesis is dependent upon L-methylfolate (shown above as MTHF), which is formed from synthetic folic acid dietary supplements, from natural dietary dihydrofolate (green vegetables, liver, etc.) or provided by direct treatment with synthetic L-methylfolate (MTHF) itself. In depressed patients, conversion of folate/folic acid into MTHF can be reduced by poor diet (e.g., alcoholism, eating disorder), by concomitant treatment with anticonvulsants that can interfere with absorption (e.g., valproic acid, carbamazepine) or inhibit the enzyme DHFR (dihydrofolate reductase) involved in L-methylfolate synthesis (e.g., lamotrigine), or by genetic factors/polymorphisms that can reduce the activity of the enzyme MTHFR (methylene tetrahydrofolate reductase), also involved in L-methylfolate synthesis. Since folic acid itself cannot cross the blood-brain barrier, and multiple factors may interfere with its conversion to L-methylfolate, treatment can be provided instead by giving L-methylfolate itself.

How Does L-methylfolate Work? Part 2:
L-methylfolate Enhances BH4 Production

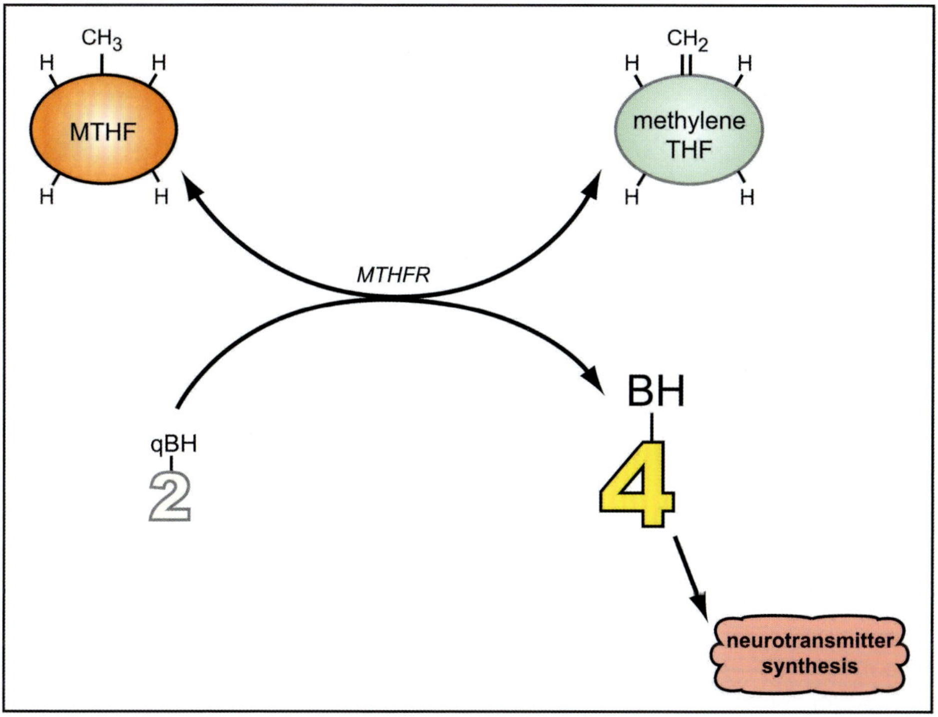

FIGURE 6.5. L-methylfolate shown as MTHF (5-methyl-tetrahydrofolate) enhances the synthesis of BH4 (tetra-hydro-biopterin). BH4 is a critical cofactor for the rate limiting enzymes that synthesize all three monoamines for trimonoamine neurotransmitter synthesis.

How Does L-methylfolate Work? Part 3:

By Enhancing BH4 Production, Boosts Trimonoamine Synthesis

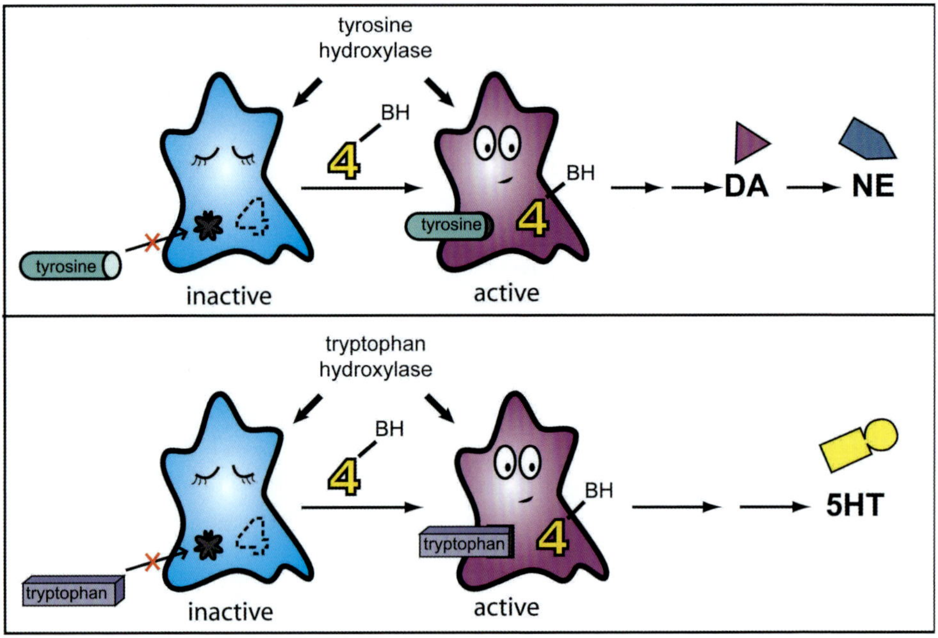

FIGURE 6.6. The rate limiting enzyme for dopamine (DA) and for norepinephrine (NE) synthesis is tyrosine hydroxylase (top panel). In the absence of BH4 cofactor, tyrosine hydroxylase is inactive (left, depicted as sleeping blue enzyme). Note also that this blue enzyme lacks BH4 binding (depicted as an empty 4) and that it cannot bind tyrosine (depicted as a stellate binding site that does not fit the round tyrosine icon). However, when BH4 binds to tyrosine hydroxylase, it "activates" the enzyme (depicted as turning purple when the yellow 4 binds as cofactor), leading to a change in the stellate binding site to a round shape in the purple enzyme. Now tyrosine can bind and be converted into both DA and NE. A similar action occurs at tryptophan hydroxylase, the rate limiting enzyme for serotonin (5HT; 5-hydroxytryptamine synthesis) (bottom).

L-methylfolate as a Trimonoamine Modulator

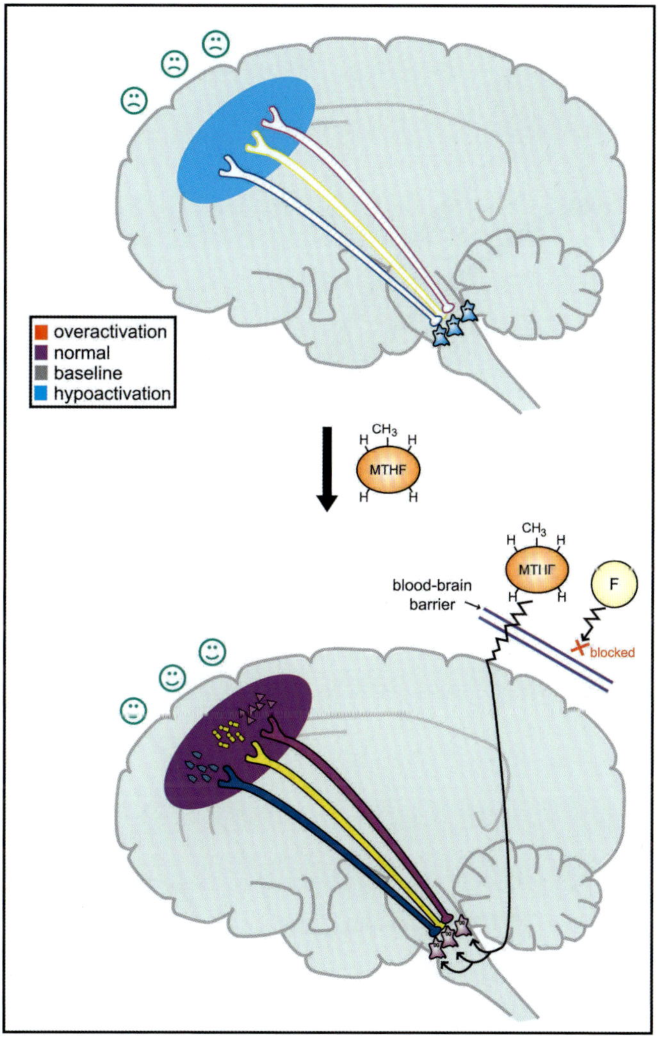

FIGURE 6.7. L-methylfolate enhances the synthesis of all three trimonoamines (dopamine, norepinephrine and serotonin), and thus is another type of TMM. Patients who are theoretically deficient in one or more of the monoamines (top; see Figs. 1.9B, 6.2 and 6.3), despite treatment with an antidepressant, can have their monoamine activity theoretically restored when L-methylfolate is added (bottom).

Neuromodulation as a Trimonoamine Modulator: Part 1

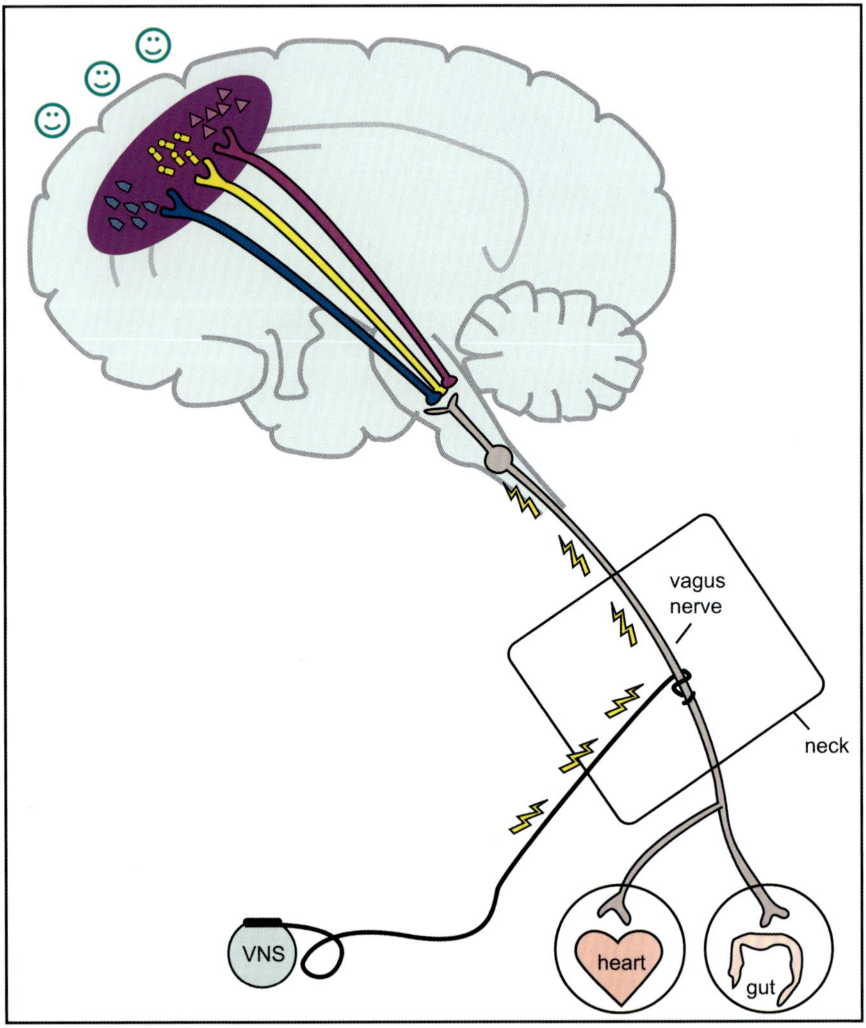

FIGURE 6.8. Stimulation of specific areas of the brain appears to be a useful therapy for difficult-to-treat depression. Vagus nerve stimulation (VNS) and deep brain stimulation (DBS, see Fig. 6.10) both utilize implanted devices in the chest wall. In VNS, a lead is wrapped around the vagus nerve in the neck. This then sends signal pulses to the midbrain raphe and locus coeruleus, thereby boosting monoamines 5HT and NE, respectively.

Neuromodulation as a Trimonoamine Modulator:

Parts 2 and 3, Transcranial Magnetic Stimulation and Deep Brain Stimulation

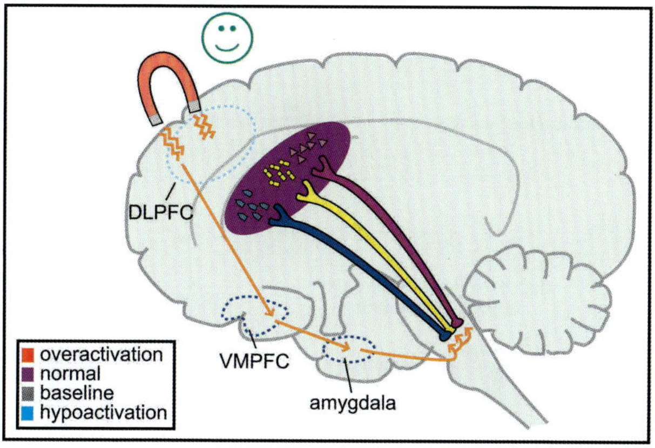

FIGURE 6.9. Transcranial magnetic stimulation (TMS) involves a coil placed on the scalp which sends magnetic stimulation specifically to the DLPFC (dorsolateral prefrontal cortex). This may boost trimonoamine neurotransmitter synthesis and release, thereby improving depressed symptoms. TMS is approved for treatment-resistant depression.

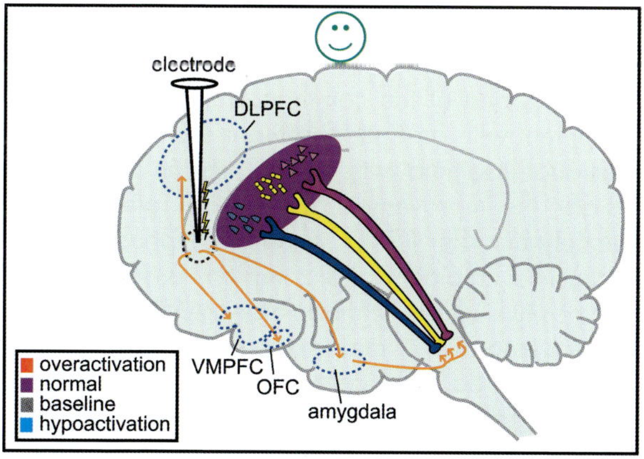

FIGURE 6.10. Deep brain stimulation (DBS) places leads directly into the brain, often in the ventromedial prefrontal cortex (VMPFC) and subgenual area of the anterior cingulate cortex (ACC). An implanted electrical stimulator sends repeated pulses and can theoretically boost the synthesis of release of the three monoamines.

Augmenting an SSRI with a "Z-Drug" Hypnotic

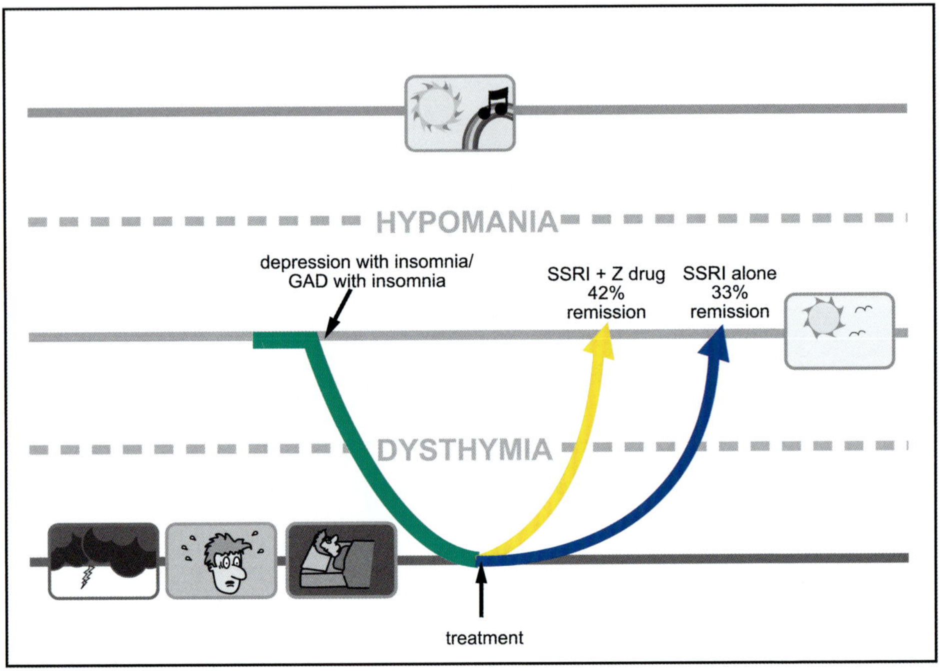

FIGURE 6.11. Insomnia is one of the commonest symptoms of major depression to persist following treatment with an antidepressant such as an SSRI. Not surprisingly, treatment of such residual insomnia with a hypnotic can improve this symptom. However, shown here is also the improvement of remission rates of both major depression and generalized anxiety disorder (GAD) when the hypnotic eszopiclone is added to an SSRI. Eszopiclone, like zolpidem and zaleplon, is sometimes called a "Z-drug" or more precisely, a positive allosteric modulator (PAM) of GABA-A receptors. Here, not only does insomnia improve in major depression and GAD when eszopiclone is added to an SSRI, but so do other core symptoms of these disorders, resulting in improvement of remission rates.

The Evolving Antidepressant Actions of Atypical Antipsychotics

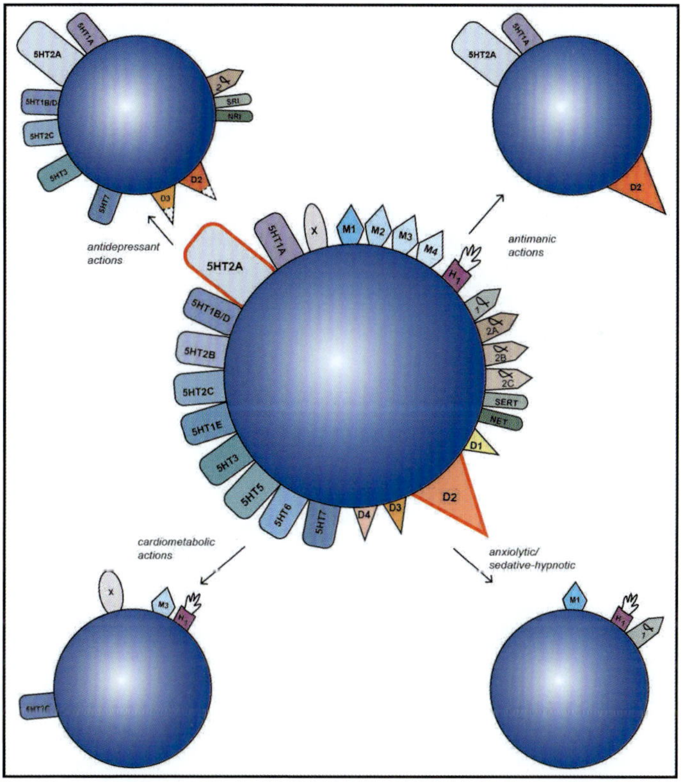

FIGURE 6.12. Atypical antipsychotics are best known as treatments of psychosis in schizophrenia and acute mania in bipolar disorder. However, these agents are increasingly being used to treat depression as well. This includes use as an augmenting agent to SSRIs or SNRIs for patients with major depression who have inadequate responses to first-line monotherapy, i.e., for treatment-resistant unipolar depression. Aripiprazole and quetiapine are currently approved by the FDA for this use, but it is likely that other agents in this class can be used as augmenting agents in treatment-resistant unipolar depression. Atypical antipsychotics are also employed both as first-line treatments for bipolar depression and as augmenting agents to mood stabilizers for bipolar depression. Quetiapine is currently approved by the FDA for this use, but all atypical antipsychotics are used in bipolar depression.

New Antidepressant Treatments on the Horizon:

Triple Reuptake Inhibitors (TRIs)

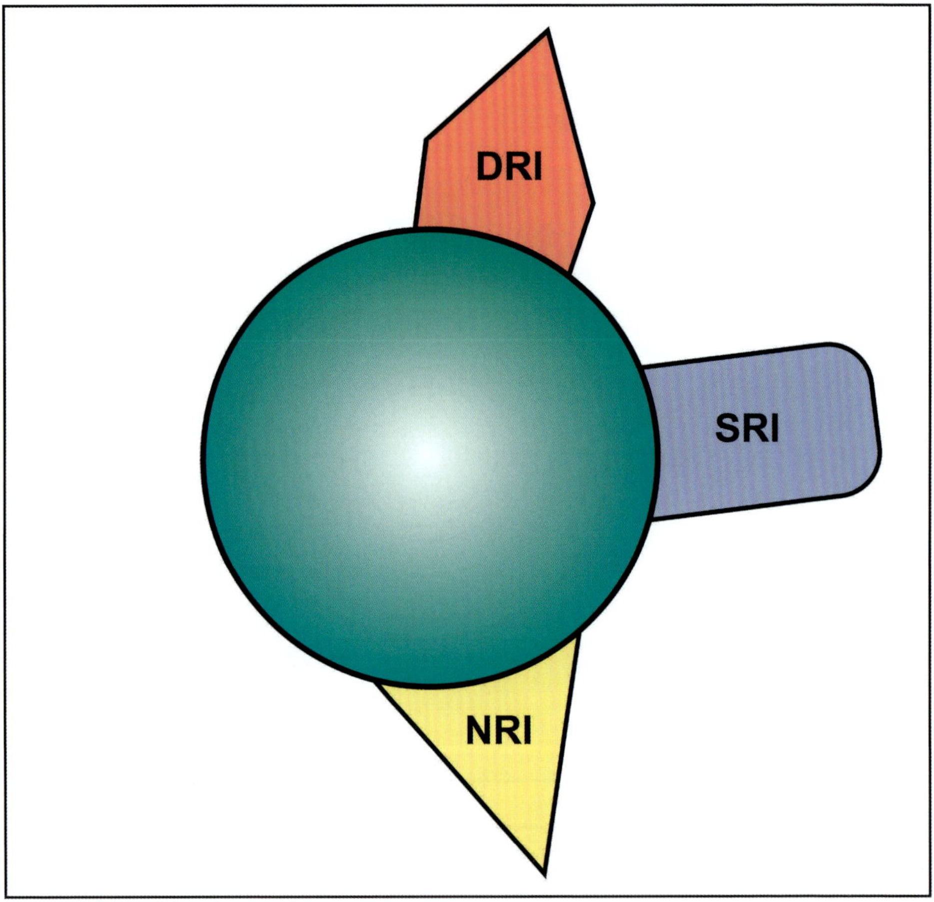

FIGURE 6.13. Triple reuptake inhibitors (TRIs) block all three monoamine transporters, thus building on the concept that if "two mechanisms are better than one" (i.e., SNRIs compared to SSRIs), then "three mechanisms may be better than two" (i.e., TRIs compared to SNRIs). At this point, the question is how much blockade of each of the three monoamine transporters would be ideal, and several of these agents are now in clinical trials. Some TRIs are in testing that have actions at multiple additional neurotransmitter receptors as well.

New Antidepressant Treatments on the Horizon:
Agomelatine

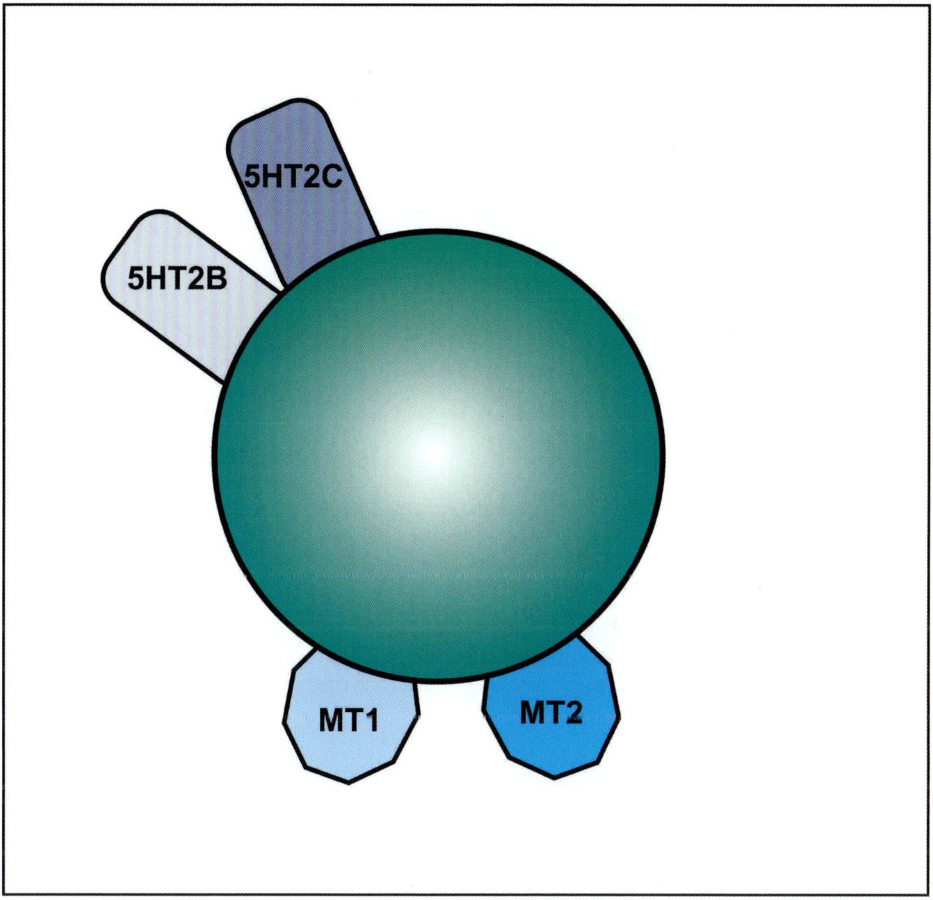

FIGURE 6.14. Agomelatine is known as a norepinephrine dopamine disinhibitor (NDDI) because of its 5HT2C antagonistic properties of inhibiting 5HT, thereby disinhibiting DA and NE release. In addition to its 5HT2C antagonist properties, agomelatine is also an agonist at melatonin 1 and melatonin 2 receptors and has 5HT2B antagonist properties. Thus, in addition to being useful in treating depression due to 5HT2C antagonist properties, its actions at MT1 and MT2 receptors can aid in sleep improvement. This agent is available in Europe.

Human Neurokinins

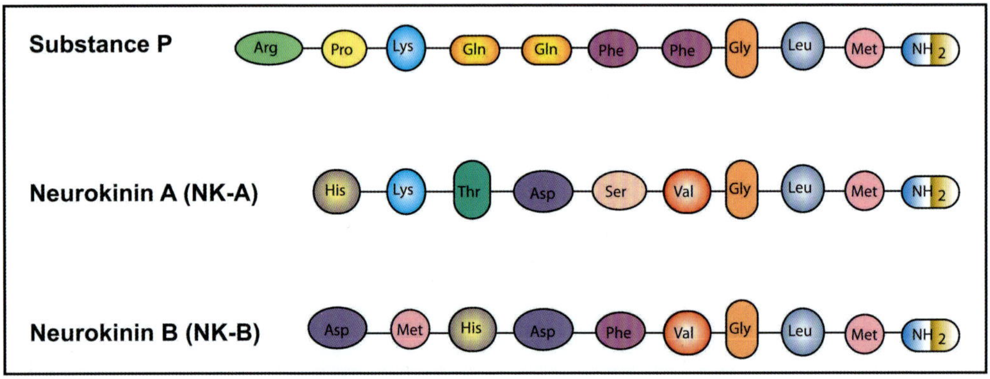

FIGURE 6.15. Amino acid sequence of the three neurokinins.

Neurokinin 1 receptors

Also called substance P receptors

Agonist is substance P

Multiple substance P antagonists (also known as NK1 antagnists) tested and failed in depression and pain

Neurokinin 2 receptors

Agonist is NKA (neurokinin A, and its extended and shortened versions)

Antagonist is saredutant, with preclinical evidence and preliminary clinical evidence of efficacy as an antidepressant

Neurokinin 3 receptors

Agonist is NKB (neurokinin B)

Multiple NK3 antagonists in testing for depression, schizophrenia and other disorders

TABLE 6.2. There are three major neurokinins in the brain: substance P (also known as neurokinin 1 or NK1), neurokinin A and neurokinin B. These are peptide neurotransmitters. There are three corresponding receptors for the neurokinins, namely NK1 receptors for substance P, NK2 receptors for neurokinin A, and NK3 receptors for neurokinin B. Currently, an NK2 receptor antagonist, saredutant, is in clinical trials (see Fig. 6.16).

New Antidepressant Treatments on the Horizon:
Saredutant, a Neurokinin 2 Antagonist

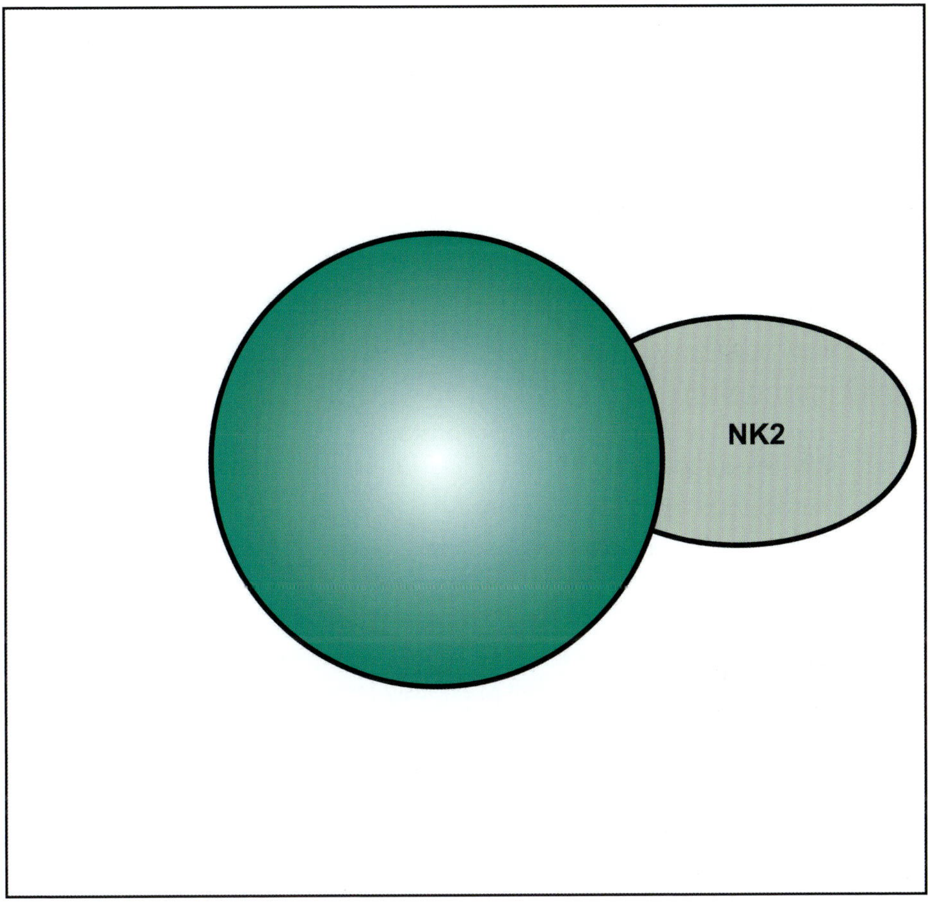

FIGURE 6.16. Saredutant, an NK2 antagonist, may be effective in patients with major depressive episodes. This agent has shown promising results in animal models of depression. Hypothetically, conditions associated with excessive release of endogenous NK-A (neurokinin A) benefit from blocking NK2 receptors; this may explain saredutant's potential antidepressant effect.

Other New Antidepressants on the Horizon

Monoamine mechanisms
5HT1A partial agonists (gepirone)
Beta 3 agonist (amebegron)
D3/D2 partial agonists (RGH-188/cariprazine; pramipexole; ropinirole; aripiprazole)
Glutamate mechanisms
Ketamine
Memantine
NMDA antagonists
Novel mechanisms
Glucocorticoid antagonists (mefipristone)
CRF1 antagonists
Vasopressin 1B (V1B) antagonists
Nemifitide (injectable pentapeptide)

TABLE 6.3. Current advances in the field of depression management. Treatment options are coming to light for MDD that previously may not have been considered for use. Some of the agents listed above were discussed in this chapter. Please refer to Stahl's Essential Psychopharmacology, 3rd ed. for further detail.

Stahl's Illustrated | Chapter 7

Depression in Women: Treating Symptoms Throughout the Life Span

This chapter focuses on women's mental health issues as they relate to depression. Specifically, women are at more risk than men for developing depression throughout their lifetimes, especially during their childbearing years. The incidence of depression in women rises during puberty. High-risk periods for onset or recurrence of a major depressive episode include the postpartum period and the perimenopausal transition to menopause. This chapter discusses how fluctuations of estrogen levels may be linked to the onset or recurrence of a major depressive episode in a woman, and provides some tips for how to manage depression in women, including evolving findings about treatment of vasomotor symptoms associated with the onset or recurrence of depression during perimenopause.

Rates of Depression Across the Life Span:
Men vs. Women

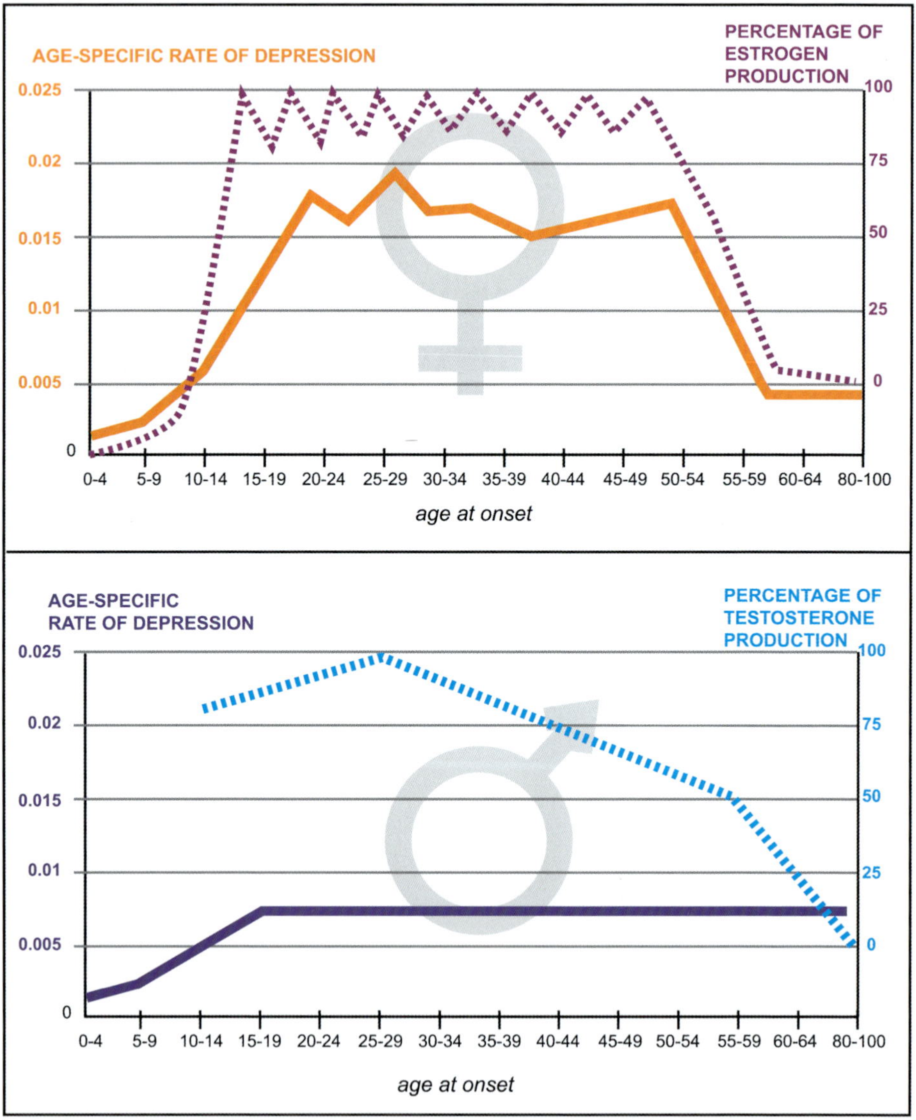

FIGURE 7.1. The rates of depression among women (top) and men (bottom) across the life span. In women, there is a link with estrogen, but in men there is no established link with testosterone.

Depression and the Link to Fluctuating Estrogen Levels Across the Female Life Cycle

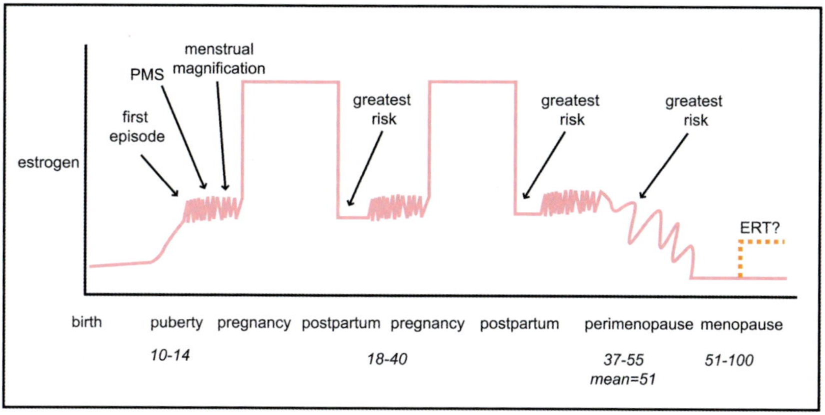

FIGURE 7.2. Postpartum and perimenopausal periods indicate the highest risk of depression for women across the life span. These periods correspond with the times of greatest fluctuations of estrogen levels across the life span.

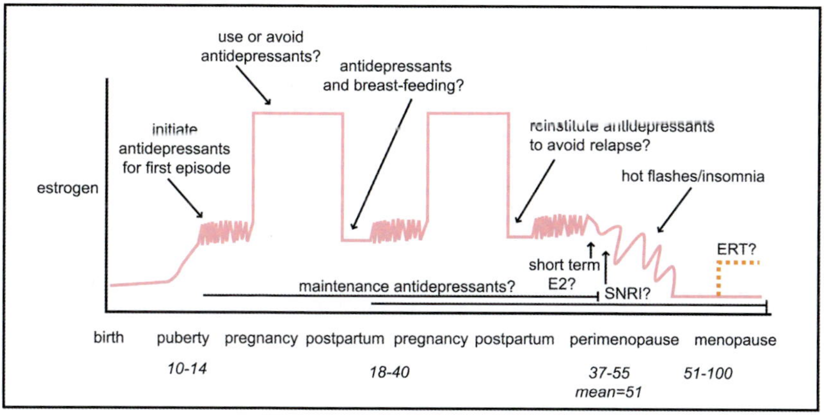

FIGURE 7.3. Pharmacotherapy use (including antidepressants and/or estrogen over the female life cycle) may vary based on the time/age of administration. Illustrated above are some of the issues that may arise in treating depression in women.

E2: estradiol. ERT: estrogen replacement therapy. SNRI: serotonin norepinephrine reuptake inhibitor.

Risks of Antidepressant Use or Avoidance During Pregnancy

Risks If You Do Treat with Antidepressants During Pregnancy

- Congenital cardiac malformations (especially first trimester; paroxetine)
- Newborn persistent pulmonary hypertension (third trimester; SSRIs)
- Neonatal withdrawal syndrome (third trimester; SSRIs)
- Prematurity, low birth weight
- Long-term neurodevelopmental abnormalities
- Increased suicidality due to antidepressant use (up to age 25)
- Medical-legal risks of using antidepressants

Risks If You Don't Treat with Antidepressants During Pregnancy

- Relapse of major depression
- Increased suicidality due to antidepressant non-use
- Poor self care
- Poor motivation for prenatal care
- Disruption of maternal-infant bonding
- Low birth weight, developmental delay in children of women with untreated depression
- Self harm
- Harm to infant
- Medical-legal risks of not using antidepressants

TABLE 7.1. Risks of treating vs. not treating women for depression during pregnancy. Clinicians are best advised to follow the literature closely and to assess risks and benefits for both mother and child on a case-by-case basis, and to document this.

Reproductive Hormones and Synaptogenesis Across the Menstrual Cycle

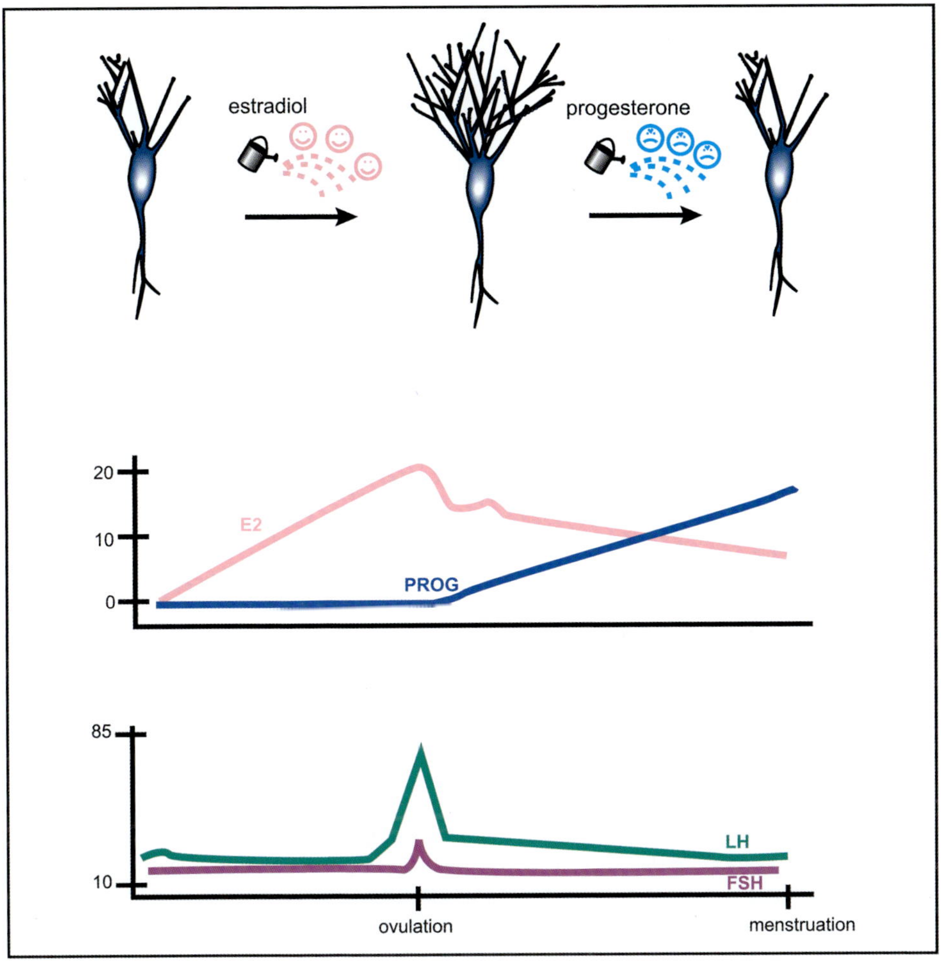

FIGURE 7.4. In the early phase of the menstrual cycle, estradiol levels rise, inducing dendritic spine formation and synaptogenesis. Progesterone peaks as well, resulting in greatest spine formation after the first half of the cycle, when estrogen is also at its highest. After this point though, estrogen levels begin to fall while progesterone continues to rise. This leads to a downregulation of dendritic spines and removal of formed synapses by the end of the menstrual cycle.

Activity-Dependent Spine Formation by Estradiol

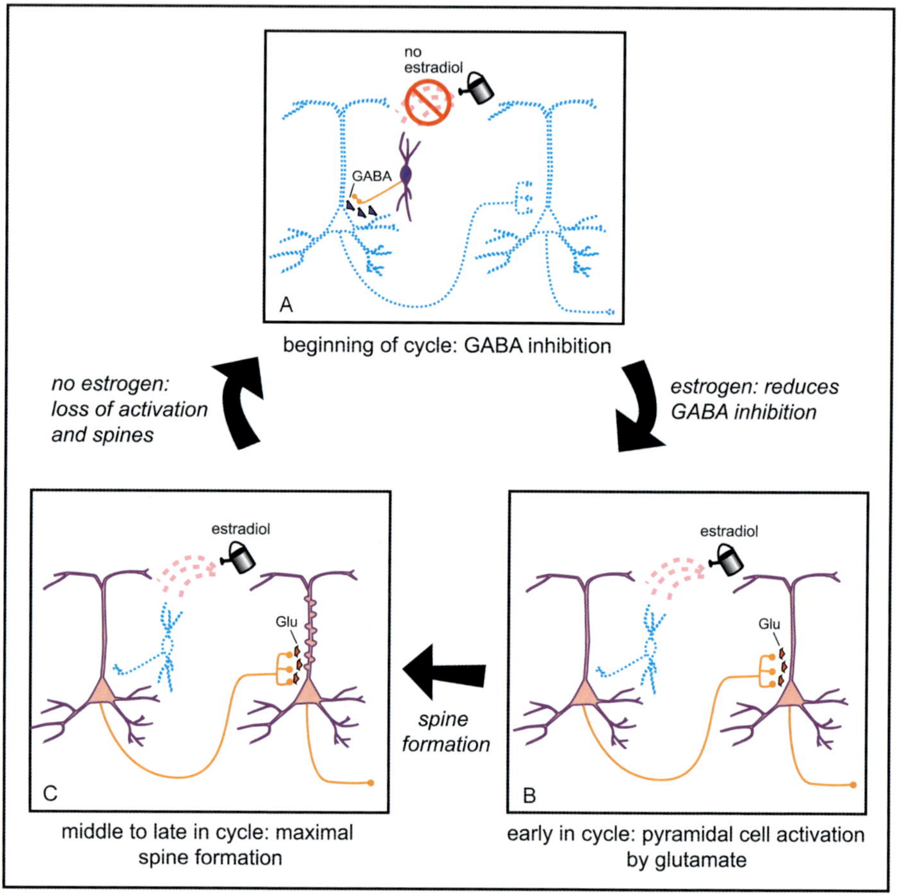

FIGURE 7.5. Estrogen exerts a cyclical inhibitory influence on gamma-aminobutyric acid (GABA) interneurons, which in turn regulate pyramidal neurons. When estrogen levels are low GABA interneurons are active and thus pyramidal neurons are inhibited (A). As estrogen levels rise early in the menstrual cycle, this reduces GABA inhibition, thus disinhibiting pyramidal neurons and leading to glutamate release (B). Sustained activation of N-methyl-d-aspartate (NMDA) receptors by glutamate, achieved by the middle or late cycle, can trigger long-term potentiation and trophic changes that include formation of dendritic spines (C). As estrogen levels fall by the end of the menstrual cycle, GABA interneurons become active again and resume inhibition of pyramidal neurons, preventing maintenance of dendritic spine formation (A).

Estrogen as a Transcription Factor

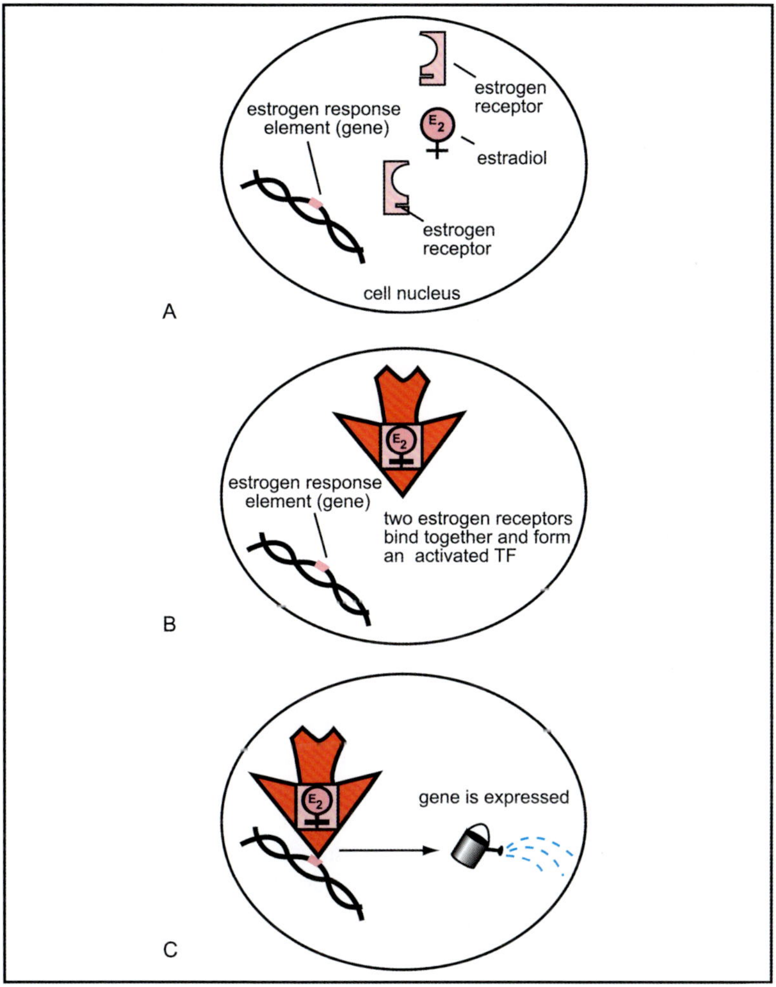

FIGURE 7.6. Estrogen binds to estrogen receptors, modulating gene expression. However, estrogen receptors differ from neurotransmitter receptors in that they are located in the neuronal cell nucleus (A). Thus, the receptor is near the gene. Estradiol activation of these genes requires dimerization of two estrogen receptors after they bind to estradiol (E2) in order to activate transcription (B). Gene products expressed by this process include nerve growth factor and brain-derived neurotrophic factor (C). Gene products also include enzymes and receptors for monoamine neurotransmitters.

Depression, Perimenopause or Both?

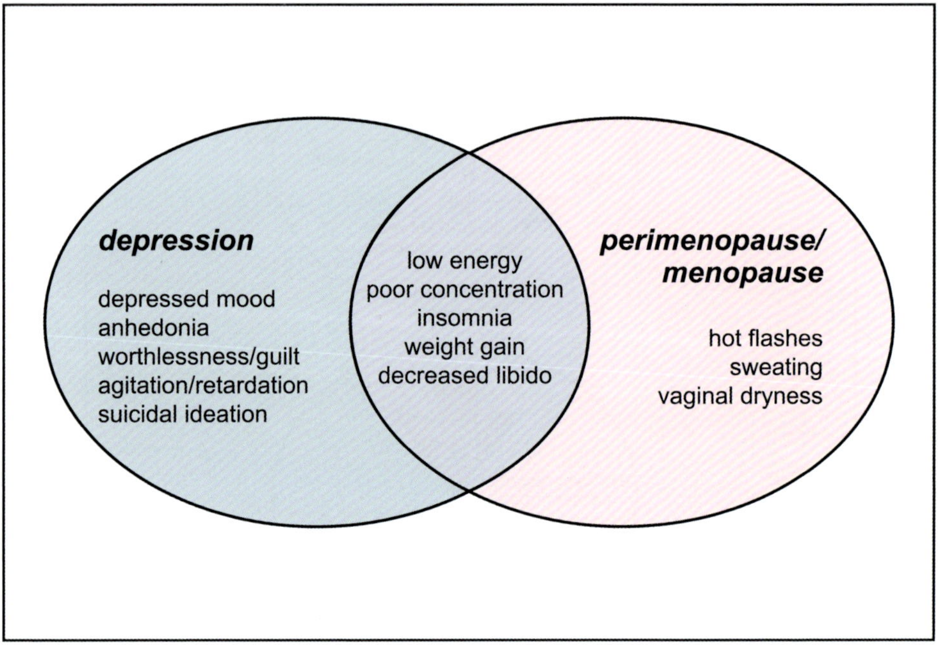

FIGURE 7.7. The clinical link between vasomotor symptoms of perimenopause/menopause and depression involves a high degree of overlapping symptoms, including low energy, poor concentration, insomnia, weight gain and decreased libido. Some experts consider vasomotor symptoms (hot flashes) as a sign of erratically fluctuating estrogen levels and not just a symptom of perimenopause, but also a risk factor for onset or recurrence of a major depressive episode in a perimenopausal woman.

Estrogen as a Trimonoamine Modulator for Vasomotor Symptoms

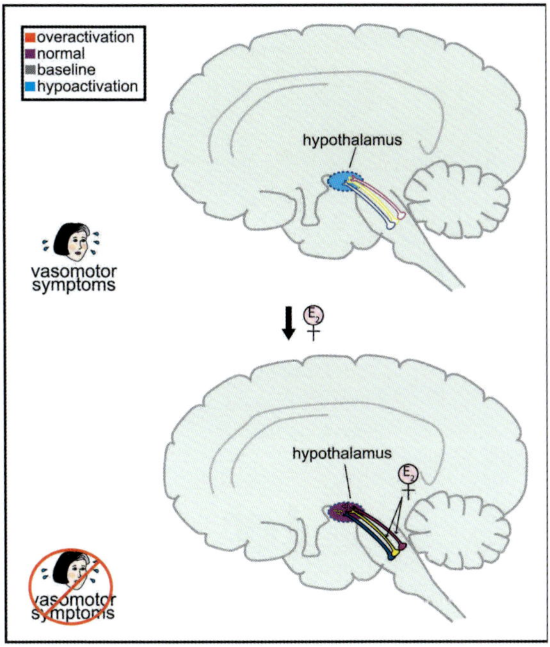

FIGURE 7.8. Vasomotor symptoms, also called hot flashes or hot flushes, are often accompanied by sweating and insomnia, all of which are well known symptoms that accompany perimenopause. Vasomotor symptoms are the clinical indication that estrogen levels are fluctuating irregularly and are increasingly recognized as the harbinger of onset or relapse of major depression during perimenopause. Fluctuating estrogen levels can theoretically create monoaminergic dysfunction in the brain. Hypothetically, dysregulation of monoaminergic control of the hypothalamic thermoregulatory centers could lead to vasomotor symptoms (top). Such patients could also hypothetically respond to the administration of estrogen with reduction of vasomotor symptoms (bottom). That is, by its effects on promoting neuronal gene expression (see Fig. 7.6), estrogen could hypothetically act as a trimonoamine modulator (TMM) (see Tab. 6.1). TMMs are discussed in chapter 6 and illustrated for lithium (see Fig. 6.2), thyroid (see Fig. 6.3) and L-methylfolate (see Fig. 6.4). Patients whose fluctuating estrogen levels cause vasomotor symptoms via dysregulation of one or more of the monoamines in hypothalamic thermoregulatory centers may restore monoamine function and thereby relieve vasomotor symptoms when given estrogen. However, many women are not willing to take estrogen for vasomotor symptoms, and most prescribers are not willing to treat long-term with estrogen due to concerns about long-term health risks. This has created the need for a non-estrogen treatment for vasomotor symptoms.

SSRIs for Vasomotor Symptoms?

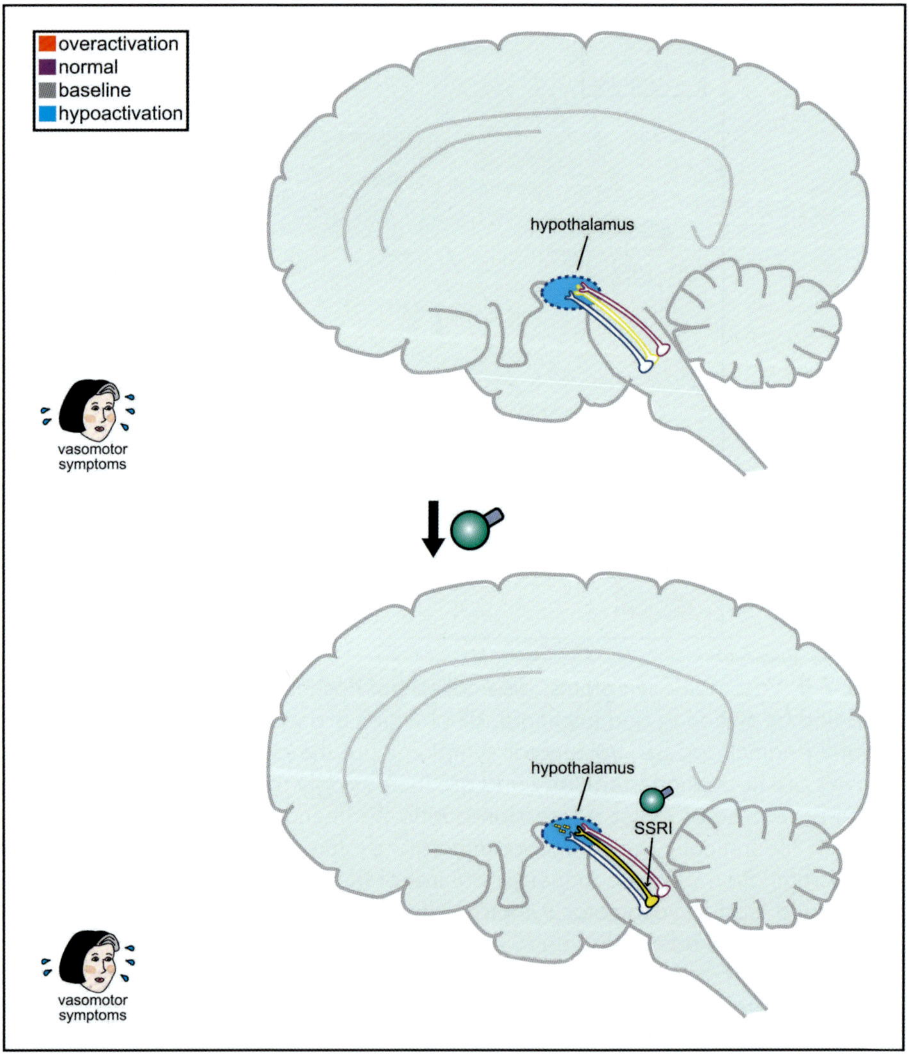

FIGURE 7.9. Vasomotor symptoms theoretically linked to fluctuating estrogen levels and causing dysregulation of monoamines in hypothalamic thermoregulatory centers. SSRIs show inconsistent benefit for vasomotor symptoms (bottom), although there are some positive results reported for paroxetine, which may in fact be a weak SNRI (see Figs. 2.14 and 7.10).

SNRIs for Vasomotor Symptoms?

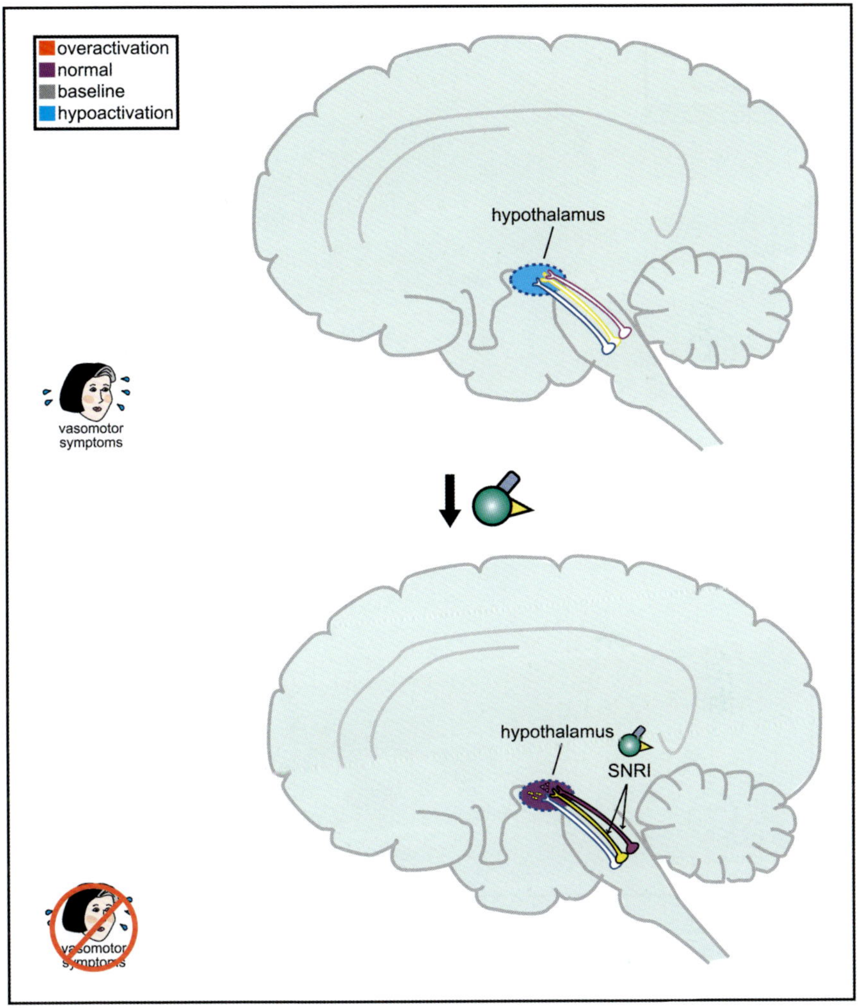

FIGURE 7.10. Vasomotor symptoms theoretically linked to fluctuating estrogen levels and causing dysregulation of monoamines in hypothalamic thermoregulatory centers are depicted at the top of this figure, as they are at the top of Figs. 7.8 and 7.9. SNRIs may show benefit for vasomotor symptoms (bottom), although such agents are not approved for this use. Under investigation is whether SNRIs have the same effect size of benefit as estrogen, and whether the benefits versus the risks of SNRIs justify their use in treating vasomotor symptoms in perimenopausal women.

Estrogen as a Trimonoamine Modulator for Depression?

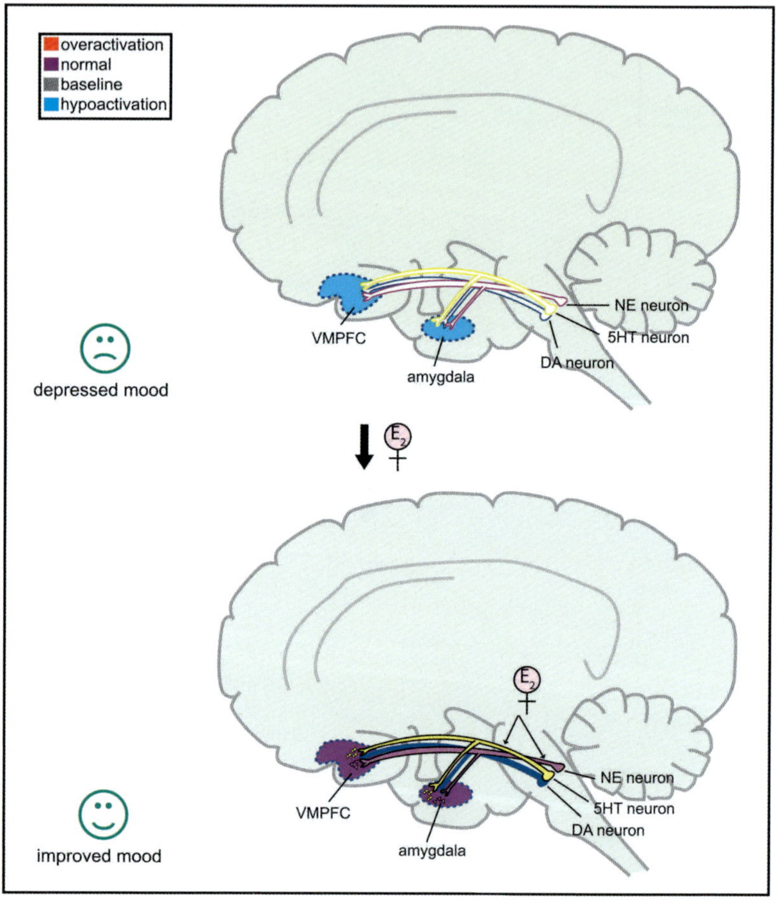

FIGURE 7.11. Estrogen can theoretically boost the actions of one or more of the three monoamines (dopamine, norepinephrine and serotonin), and thus is a trimonaomine modulator (TMM) (see Tab. 6.1 and Fig. 7.8). Patients who are theoretically deficient in one or more of the three monoamines, as may theoretically occur in women particularly in the postpartum and perimenopausal periods when estrogen levels can fluctuate widely, or in the postmenopausal period when estrogen levels are low (top; see Fig. 7.2) can have their monoamine activity theoretically restored when estrogen is added (bottom). However, this is not an approved use for estrogen, and many women and their prescribers wish to avoid estrogen use due to long-term risks to health.

SSRIs for Perimenopausal or Postmenopausal Depression?

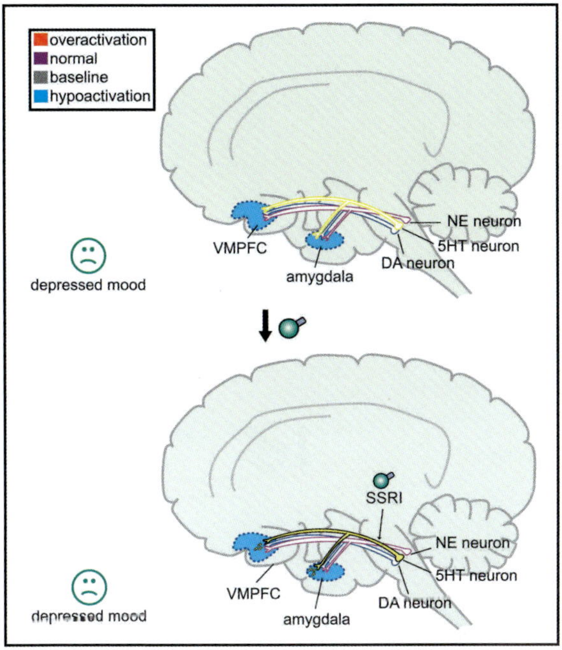

FIGURE 7.12. Due to the association of vasomotor symptoms with the onset or recurrence of a major depressive episode, experts now debate whether prescribers should identify and treat vasomotor symptoms as well as the traditional symptoms of depression in perimenopausal women. Actually, the treatments for these two conditions overlap (see Figs. 7.7 – 7.13). Treating vasomotor symptoms could theoretically prevent a major depressive episode in vulnerable women. Furthermore, failure to treat vasomotor symptoms in a perimenopausal woman who also has a major depressive episode may stand in the way of reaching full remission of the major depressive episode, or of sustaining that remission in the long run. That is, remission of the classic symptoms of depression while vasomotor symptoms persist is a likely signal that fluctuating estrogen levels are still affecting the brain and may continue to create vulnerability for relapse. Ongoing research is seeking to determine whether targeting vasomotor symptoms in women with depression or at risk for depression will achieve better outcomes. In the meantime, if SSRIs for such women are not effective (see bottom of Fig. 7.12 above and Fig. 7.9), it may be worthwhile to treat with SNRIs (see Fig. 7.10 and 7.13). Furthermore, SSRIs seem to work better in the presence of estrogen (see Figs. 7.11) than in the absence of estrogen (bottom). Thus, SSRIs may be more reliable in premenopausal women or in peri- or postmenopausal women who are taking estrogen.

SNRIs for Perimenopausal Depression?

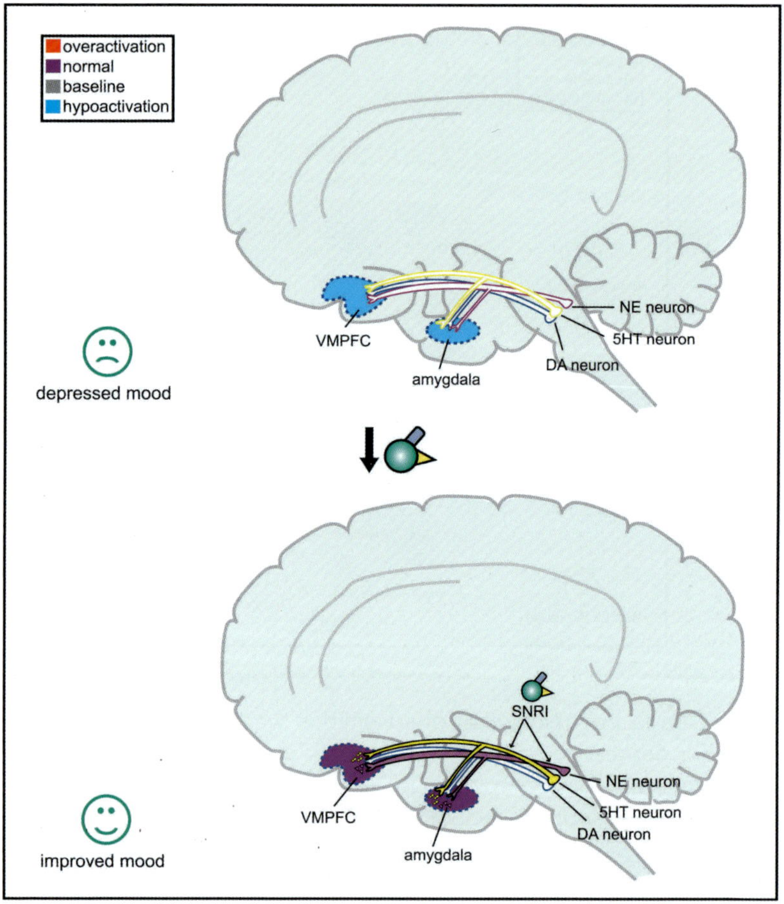

FIGURE 7.13. To treat both vasomotor symptoms and symptoms of a major depressive episode in a perimenopausal woman with fluctuating estrogen levels or in a postmenopausal woman with low estrogen levels (top), SNRIs may be preferred (bottom). There is some evidence that SNRIs can not only relieve vasomotor symptoms (see Fig. 7.10), but also treat symptoms of a major depressive episode in peri- and postmenopausal women, even if they are not taking estrogen (bottom). However, further research is in progress.

Pharmacokinetics and Algorithms to Treat Depression

Pharmacokinetics of antidepressants must be considered when choosing and combining treatments for patients. Information on drug interactions is constantly being updated. This chapter reviews the basic principles of antidepressant pharmacokinetics, but specifics are best found in up-to-date reference sources on prescribing.

Once treatment options have been investigated, algorithms to treat depression may help the clinician in deciding the best treatment choice on a per-case basis. Current algorithms that may be utilized in the treatment of depression can be evidence-based, cost-based or symptom-based. Whereas evidence- and cost-based algorithms may be more beneficial to healthcare plans in terms of financial issues, patients often benefit most from a symptom-based approach. This may require some trial and error, but once the correct treatment option is chosen, patients may experience complete remission of depressive symptoms. Whatever approach is taken, the goal of treatment of depression is remission. Here, we emphasize the symptom-based approach to selecting and combining antidepressants, particularly for difficult cases.

Pharmacokinetics of Antidepressants: CYP450

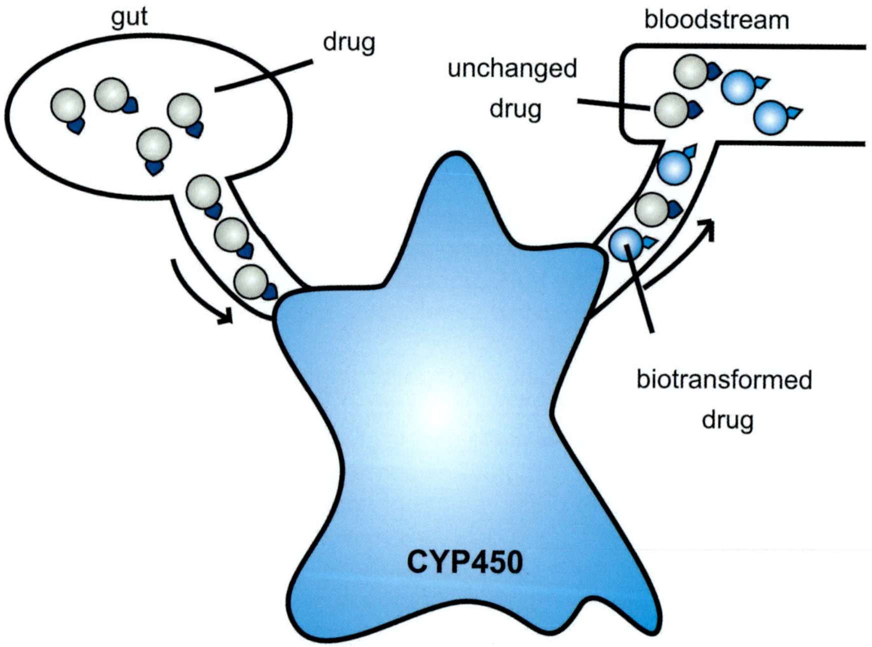

FIGURE 8.1. The cytochrome P450 (CYP450) enzyme system, which is located in the gut wall and liver, is responsible for the way the body metabolizes drugs such as antidepressants. When the drug substrate passes through the gut, it is biotransformed into a product released into the bloodstream. Thus upon administration, a drug is partially metabolized by the CYP450 system and partially left unchanged.

Specifics of the CYP450 System

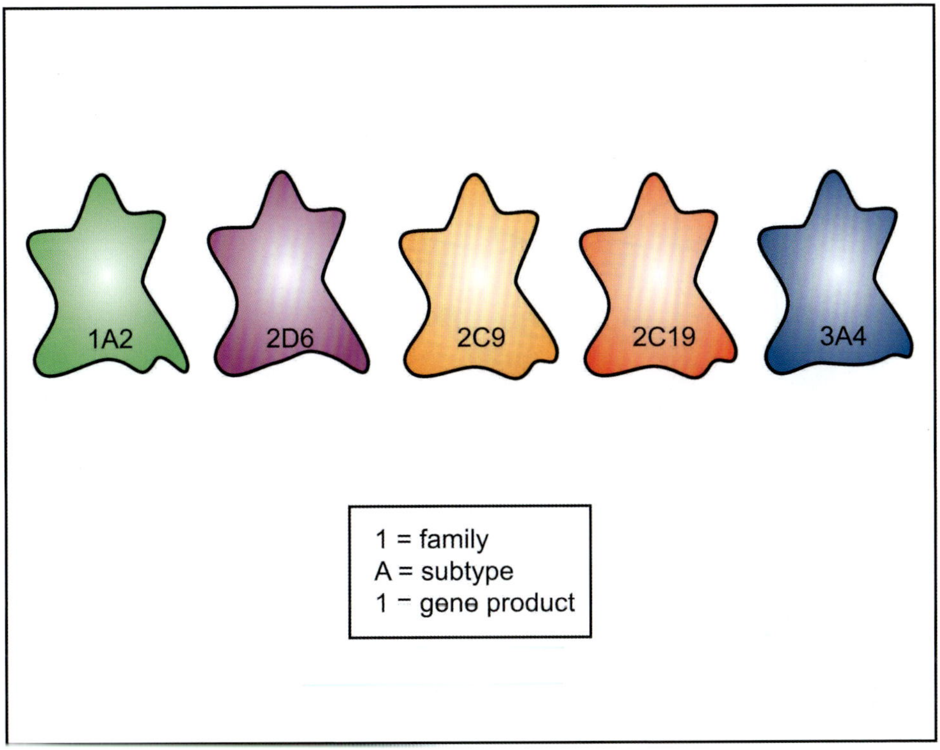

FIGURE 8.2. The cytochrome P450 system encompasses a large number of enzymes. These are classified according to family, subtype, and gene product, using the following nomenclature: 1= family, A=subtype, and 1=gene product. Thus, as depicted in the figure, the five most common and relevant systems are CYP450 1A2, 2D6, 2C9, 2C19, and 3A4.

Genetic Polymorphism for CYP450 2D6

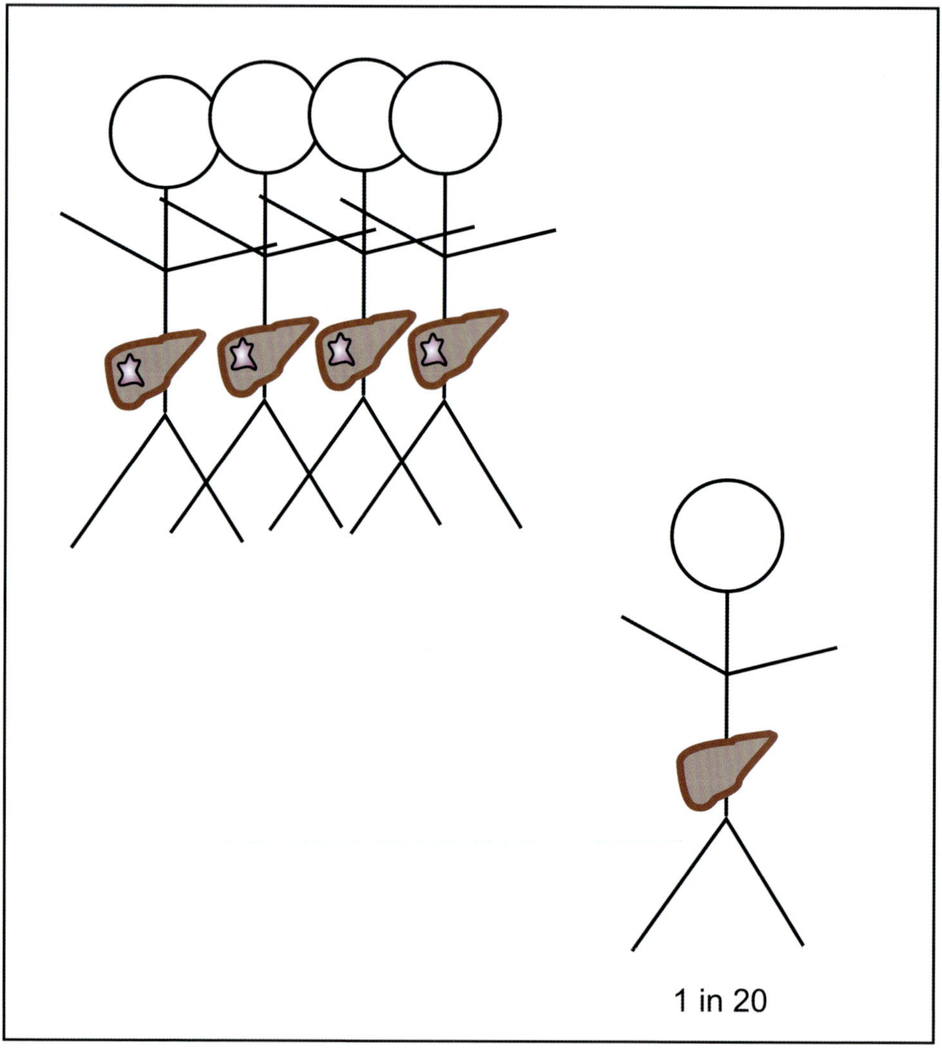

FIGURE 8.3. An individual's genetic make-up determines which CYP450 enzymes s/he has. For example, approximately 1 in 20 Caucasians is a poor metabolizer via 2D6 and thus needs to metabolize drugs by an alternative route. This may (1) not be as metabolically efficient and (2) explain the differential efficacy of various antidepressants in different patients.

Pharmacokinetics of Antidepressants: CYP450 1A2

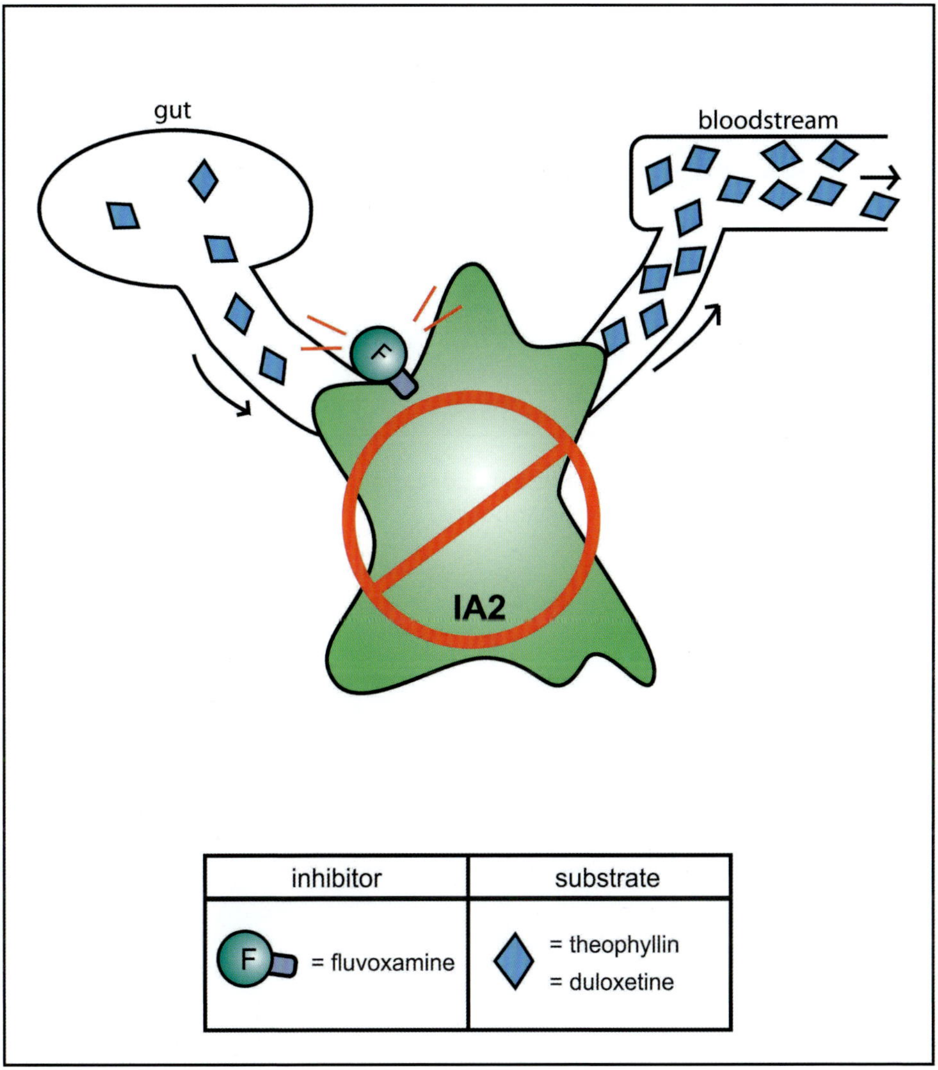

FIGURE 8.4. Substrate levels of 1A2, listed above, can rise dramatically in the presence of fluvoxamine (inhibitor of 1A2). Thus, doses must be lowered to avoid this effect.

Pharmacokinetics of Antidepressants:
CYP450 2D6

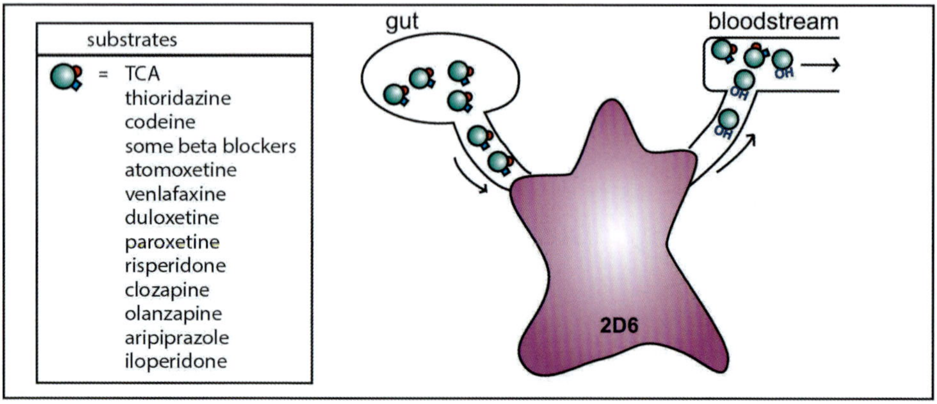

FIGURE 8.5. Some antidepressants listed above are substrates of 2D6, which converts these agents to active or inactive metabolites.

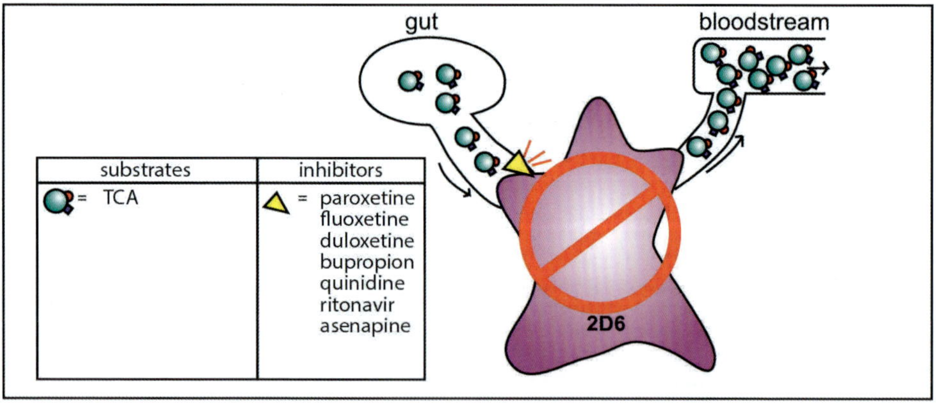

FIGURE 8.6. Tricyclic antidepressants are substrates of CYP450 2D6. Combining TCAs with SSRIs or SNRIs that inhibit 2D6 can lead to toxic levels of TCAs in the bloodstream. This can be monitored by measuring plasma drug concentration and by dose reduction as needed, if such medications are to be administered simultaneously.

Pharmacokinetics of Antidepressants:
CYP450 3A4

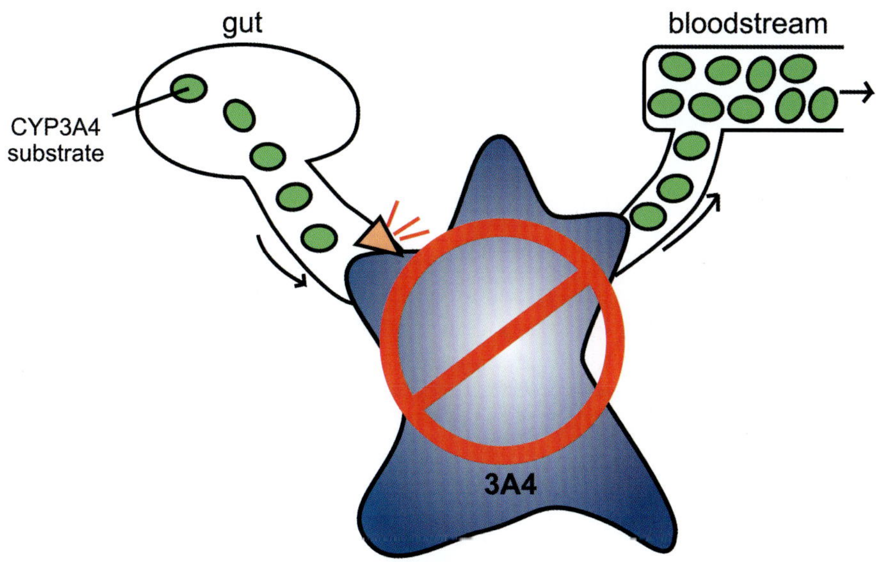

substrates	inhibitors
(green oval) = pimozide alprazolam triazolam buspirone HMG-CoA reductase inhibitors (simvastatin, atorvastatin, lovastatin, cerevastatin) clozapine quetiapine sertindole aripiprazole zotepine lurasidone iloperidone	(triangle) = fluvoxamine fluoxetine nefazodone erythromycin ketoconazole protease inhibitors verapamil diltiazem

FIGURE 8.7. Antidepressants such as fluvoxamine, fluoxetine and nefazodone are moderate inhibitors of the CYP450 3A4 enzyme, as illustrated above.

Response Rates:
Antidepressants vs. Placebo

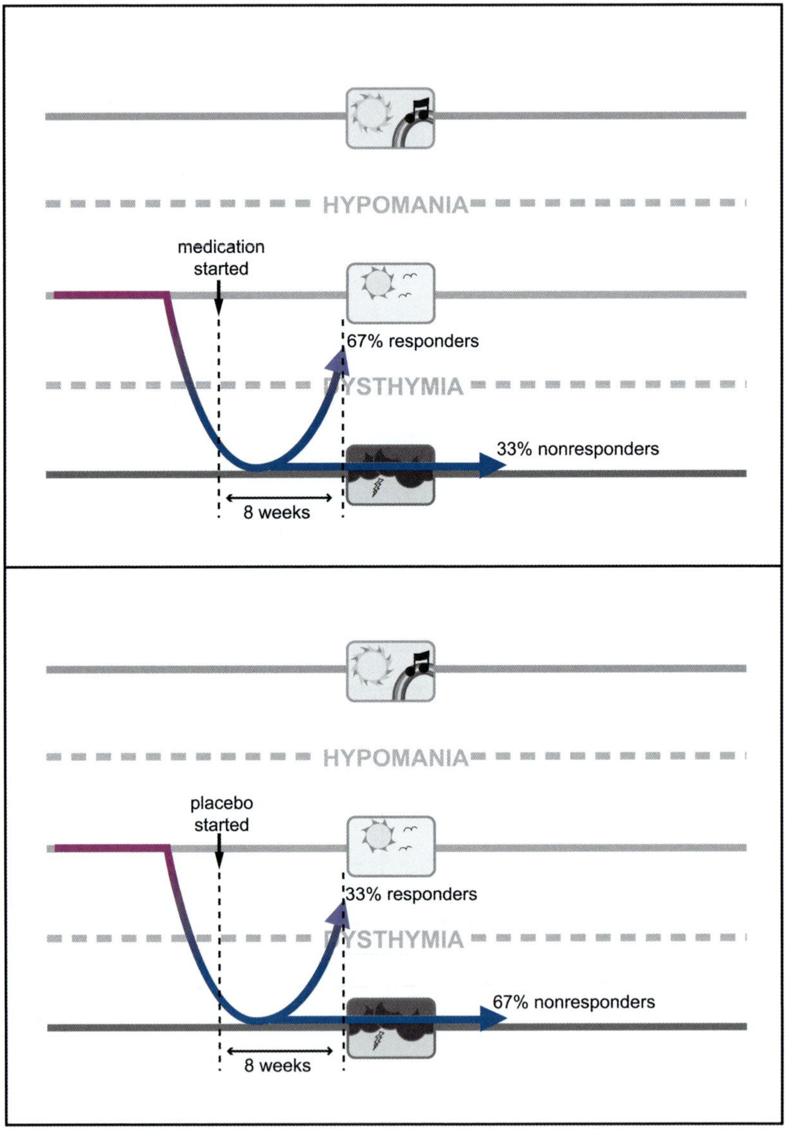

FIGURE 8.8. In 8-week clinical trials, the majority of antidepressants yield 67% responders and 33% non-responders, while a placebo results in 33% responders and 67% non-responders.

Rate of Remission in MDD vs. Residual Symptoms in Nonremitters

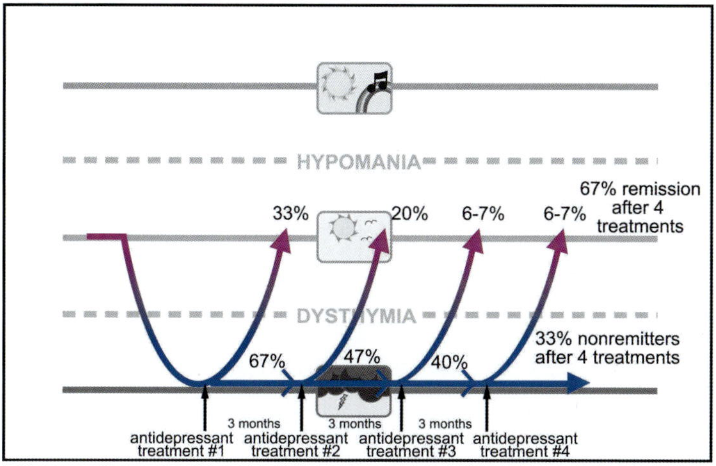

FIGURE 8.9. Only 1/3 of patients remit after initial treatment. After a year of treatment with four different antidepressants for 12 weeks each, only 2/3 of patients eventually achieve remission.

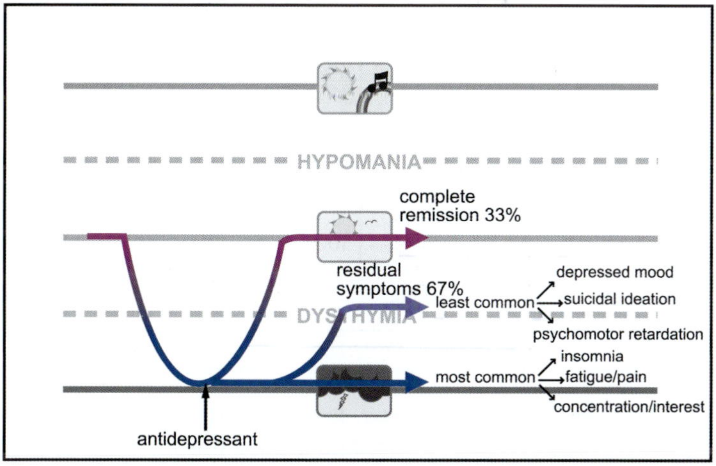

FIGURE 8.10. While antidepressants are more likely to improve mood, suicidal ideation and psychomotor retardation in depressed patients, several symptoms often remain in non-remitters, especially insomnia, but also fatigue and problems concentrating.

Proportion of MDD Relapses

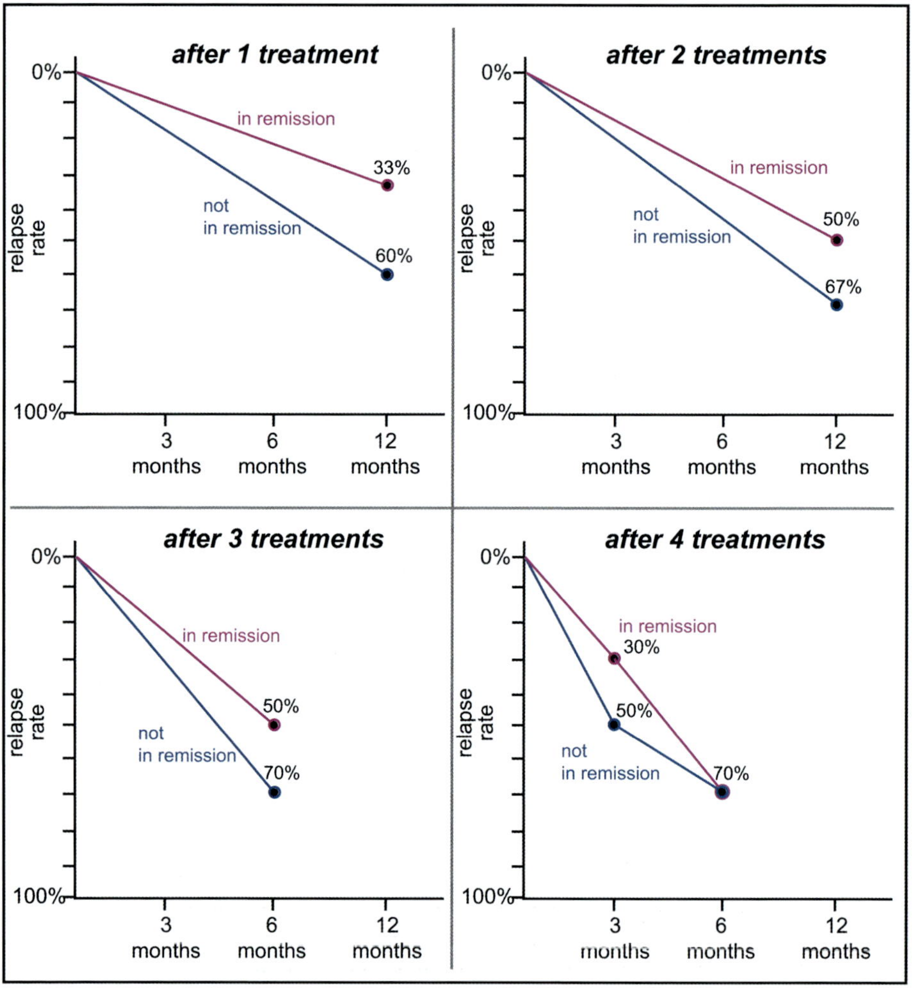

FIGURE 8.11. Once remission is achieved, there appears to be a protective factor in experiencing a relapse. However, as treatment administration increases, the protective effect of remission decreases. Thus, as shown above, a patient who achieved remission after 1 treatment has a higher rate of staying in remission, whereas a patient who remitted only after 4 treatments has a much lower rate of staying in remission. Furthermore, the chances of staying in remission decline as the number of treatments required to attain remission increase.

Positive and Negative Affect

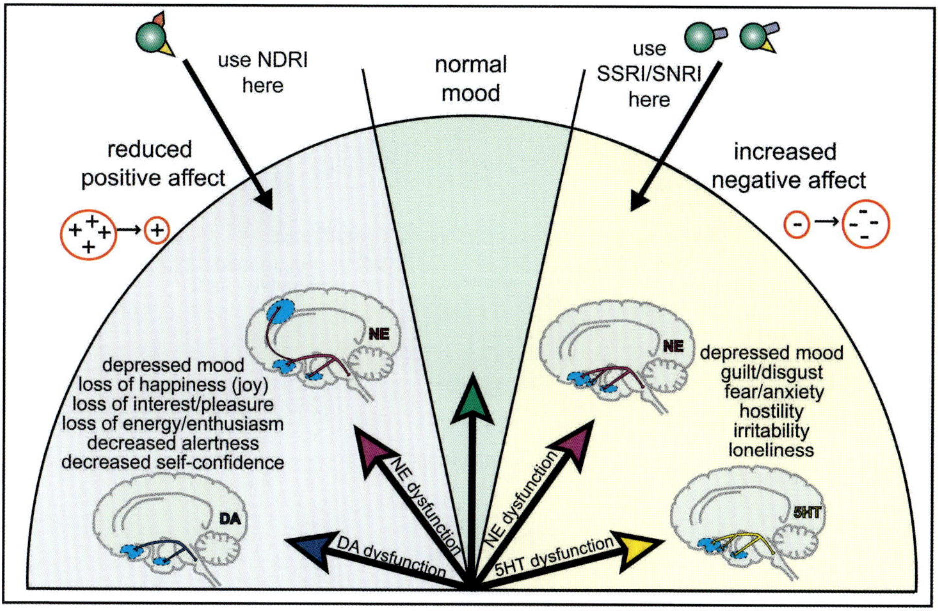

FIGURE 8.12. Mood-related symptoms of depression can be characterized by their affective expression—that is, whether they cause a reduction in positive affect or an increase in negative affect. Symptoms related to reduced positive affect include depressed mood, loss of happiness, interest, or pleasure, loss of energy or enthusiasm, decreased alertness, and decreased self-confidence. Reduced positive affect may be hypothetically related to dopaminergic dysfunction, with a possible role of noradrenergic dysfunction as well. Such patients may respond best to antidepressants that boost DA (and NE) (see Fig. 8.13). Symptoms associated with increased negative affect include depressed mood, guilt, disgust, fear, anxiety, hostility, irritability, and loneliness. Increased negative affect may be linked hypothetically to serotonergic dysfunction and perhaps also to noradrenergic dysfunction. Such patients may respond best to antidepressants that boost 5HT (and NE) (see Fig. 8.13).

Symptom-Based Algorithm for Positive and Negative Affect

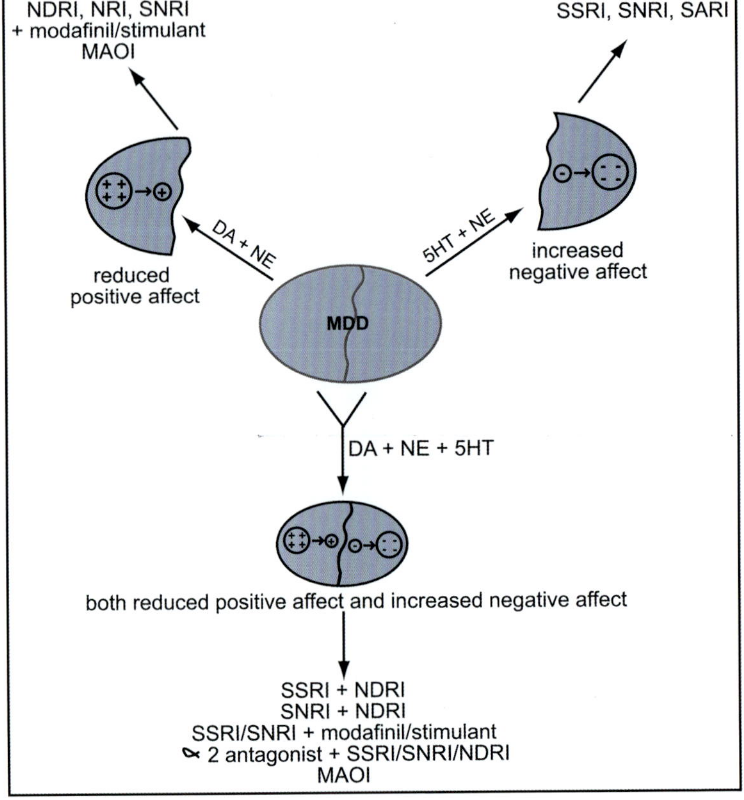

FIGURE 8.13. The symptom-based treatment algorithm is based on treating symptoms that match the circuits and neurotransmitters that hypothetically mediate them. Thus, knowing whether the patient is experiencing reduced positive affect or increased negative affect, or both, is an integral part of the treatment process. Specific antidepressant monotherapies and combinations are suggested that are unique for treating reduced positive affect, increased negative affect, or both.

MDD: major depressive disorder. NDRI: norepinephrine and dopamine reuptake inhibitors. NRI: norepinephrine reuptake inhibitors. SSRI: selective serotonin reuptake inhibitors. SNRI: serotonin norepinephrine reuptake inhibitors. SARI: serotonin antagonist/reuptake inhibitors. MAOI: monoamine oxidase inhibitors. 5HT: serotonin. NE: norepinephrine. DA: dopamine.

Symptom-Based Treatment Algorithm for Depression

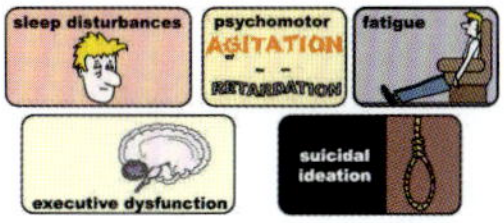

Step 1: Identify diagnostic and associated symptoms

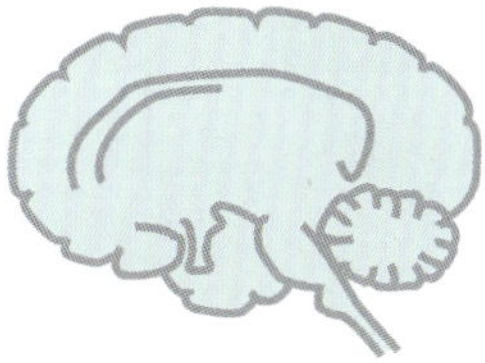

Step 2: Match symptom to malfunctioning brain circuit

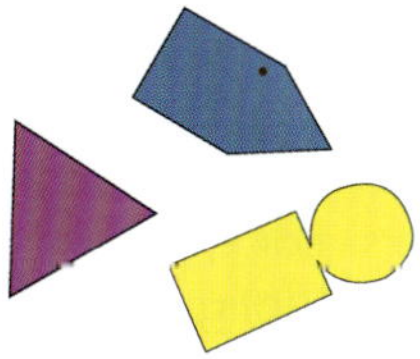

Step 3: Target specific neurotransmitters and pharmacologic mechanisms

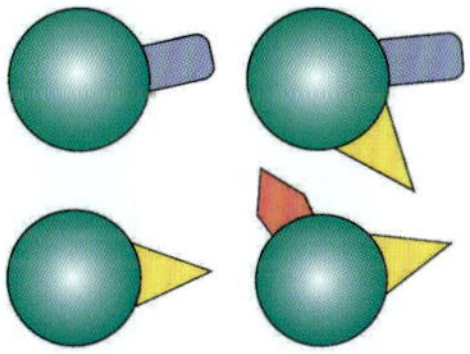

Step 4: Match malfunction to pharmacologic mechanism

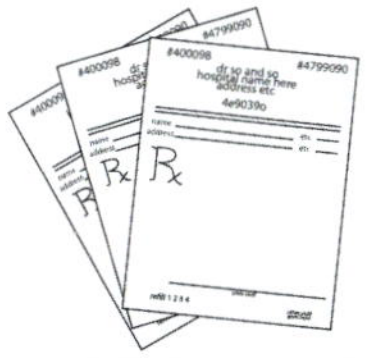

Step 5: Construct unique treatment portfolio for one patient at a time

FIGURE 8.14. Although this is a highly simplified explanation for treating a complex disorder that involves a variety of interacting brain regions, the concept of personalizing treatment plans for unique sets of symptoms is an important one.

Symptom-Based Algorithm for Antidepressants: Parts 1 and 2

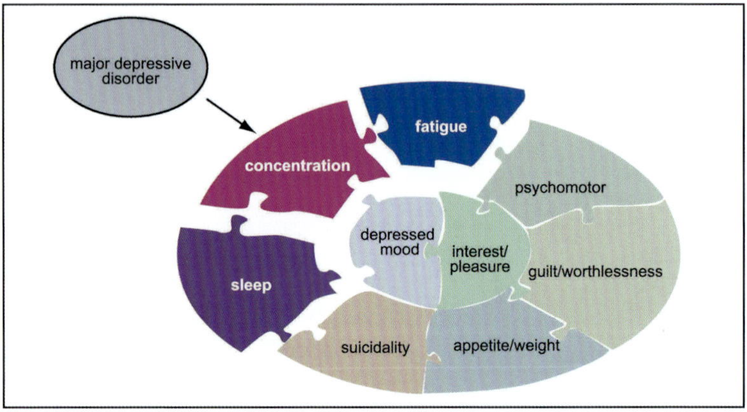

FIGURE 8.15. The components of a diagnosis of MDD according to the DSM-IV. The most common residual symptoms are fatigue, problems concentrating, and sleep disturbances, as also shown in Fig. 8.10. Step 1 is to deconstruct the individual patient's major depressive disorder into its specific symptom components. For example, even after initial treatment, it is common for patients to have persistent fatigue, insomnia and problems concentrating.

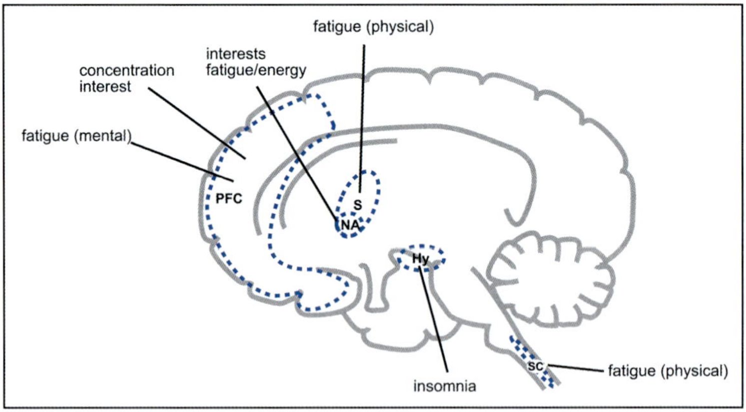

FIGURE 8.16. Step 2 is to match the most common residual symptoms to hypothetically malfunctioning brain circuits. Shown here are the hypothetical brain circuits associated with the most common residual symptoms of depression shown in Fig. 8.15.

Symptom-Based Algorithm for Antidepressants: Part 3

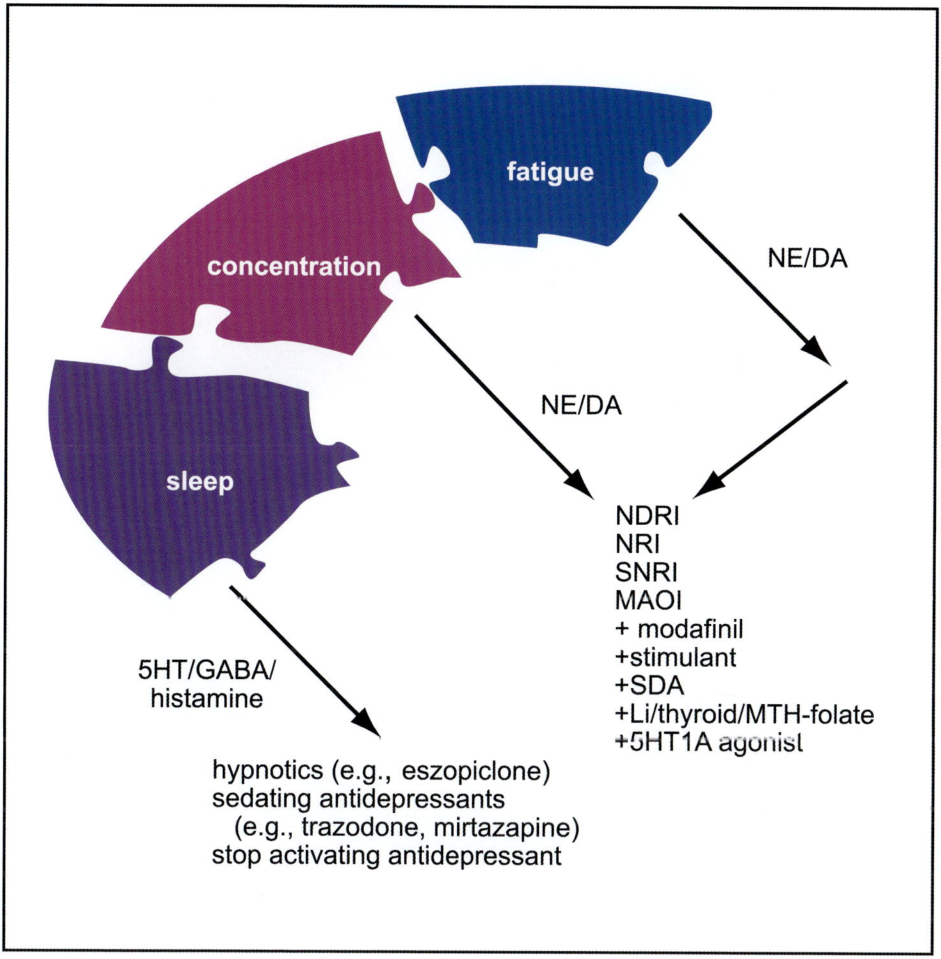

FIGURE 8.17. After deconstructing MDD into its specific symptoms and then matching them to hypothetically malfunctioning brain circuits, the clinician can move on to targeting the regulatory neurotransmitters associated with these specific brain circuits (step 3). Knowing this will allow selection of a treatment that specifically targets these neurotransmitters (step 4). Several such treatments are shown for the common residual symptoms of insomnia, fatigue and problems concentrating, and differ rationally depending upon the specific symptom. Step 5 is to construct a unique treatment portfolio targeting all symptoms of an individual patient.

Treating All 14 of the Nine Symptoms of Depression: Part 1

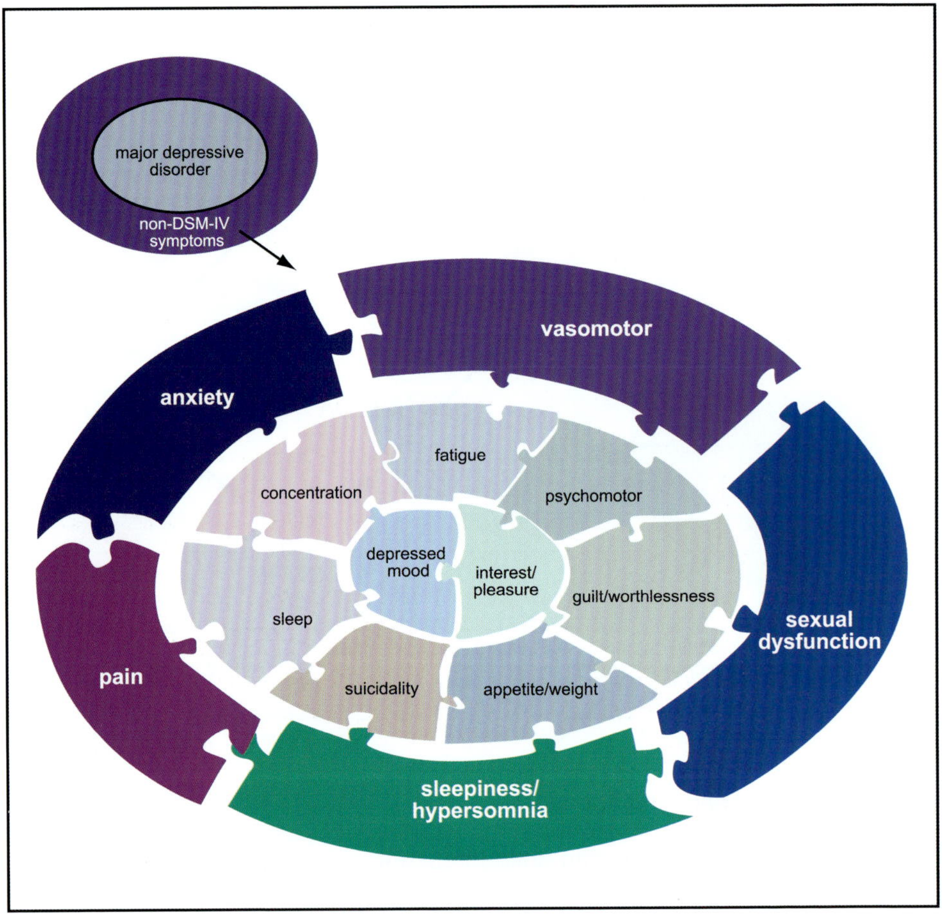

FIGURE 8.18. Additional symptoms of MDD that may not be listed in the official diagnostic criteria include pain, sleepiness, anxiety, vasomotor symptoms and sexual dysfunction. Vasomotor symptoms are discussed extensively in chapter 7 (see Figs. 7.7 – 7.13).

Treating All 14 of the Nine Symptoms of Depression: Parts 2 and 3

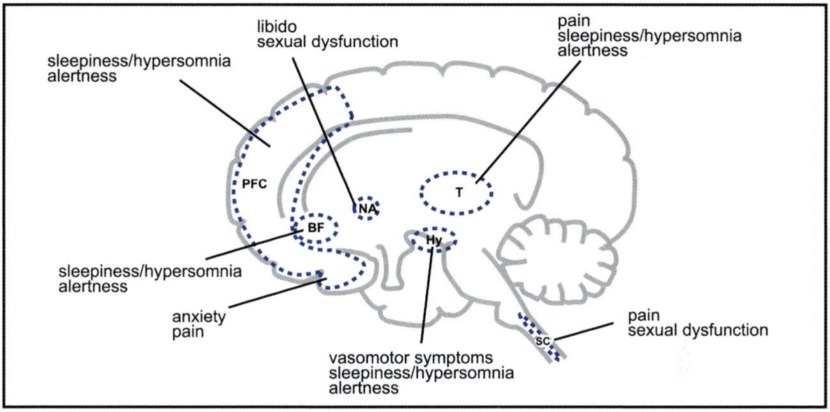

FIGURE 8.19. Matching these additional symptoms associated with MDD to hypothetically malfunctioning brain circuits can aid in determining the best course of treatment, just as discussed above for the core diagnostic symptoms of MDD.

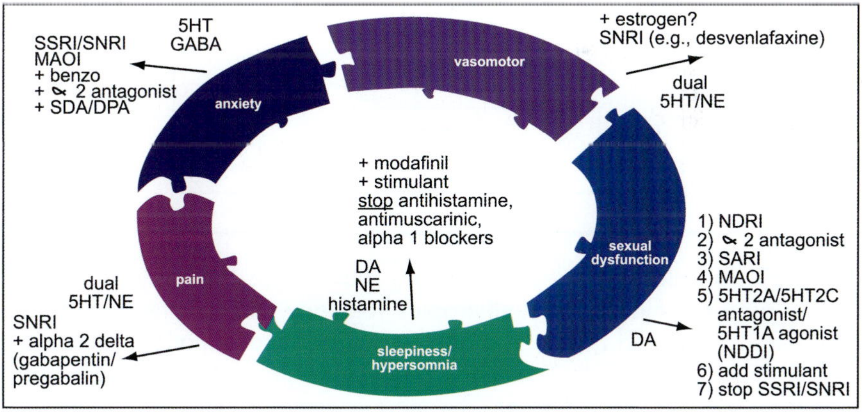

FIGURE 8.20. Treating all symptoms of depression, including those not in the official diagnosis, is important to attain a true remission and recovery. Again, targeting the regulatory neurotransmitters involved in these processes aids in understanding how to select the best treatment options for individual symptoms as shown here. Thus one should "treat all 14 of the nine symptoms of major depression" (comparing Fig. 8.18 with Fig. 8.15).

First-Line Monotherapies Followed by Classical Evidence-Based Antidepressant Augmentation Therapies

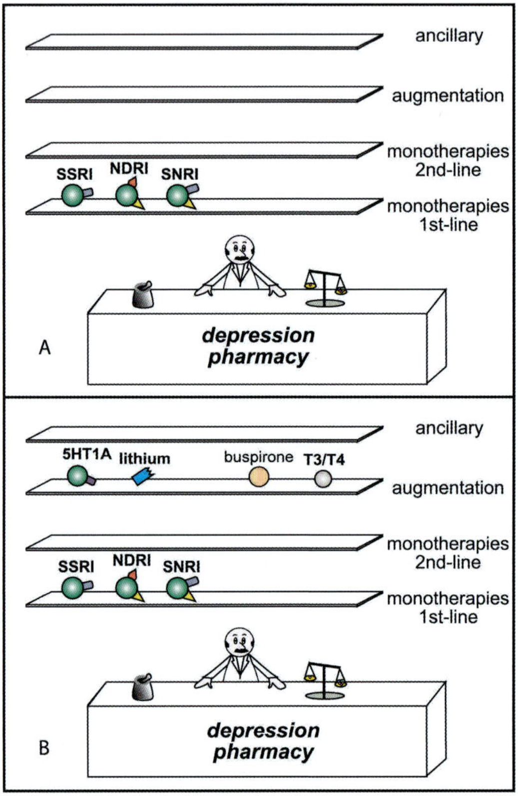

FIGURE 8.21. The algorithm depicted above shows steps that may be taken when treating depression. First-line monotherapies regularly utilized are shown (A), and include SSRIs, SNRIs and NDRIs as monotherapy or in combination with each other (e.g., SSRI/SNRI plus NDRI). This is followed by augmentation strategies (B) if the monotherapy alone is not sufficient. The most common augmentation therapies for major depression have often included lithium (see Fig. 6.2), thyroid (see Fig. 6.3) or the 5HT1A partial agonist buspirone (B). However, recent evidence-based studies do not suggest which patient should get each of these and are not able to determined which is superior to the others.

SSRI: selective serotonin reuptake inhibitors. SNRI: serotonin norepinephrine reuptake inhibitors. NDRI: norepinephrine and dopamine reuptake inhibitors. 5HT1A: serotonin 1A agonists. T3/T4: thyroid hormone.

Second-Line Monotherapies and Ancillary Treatments for Depression

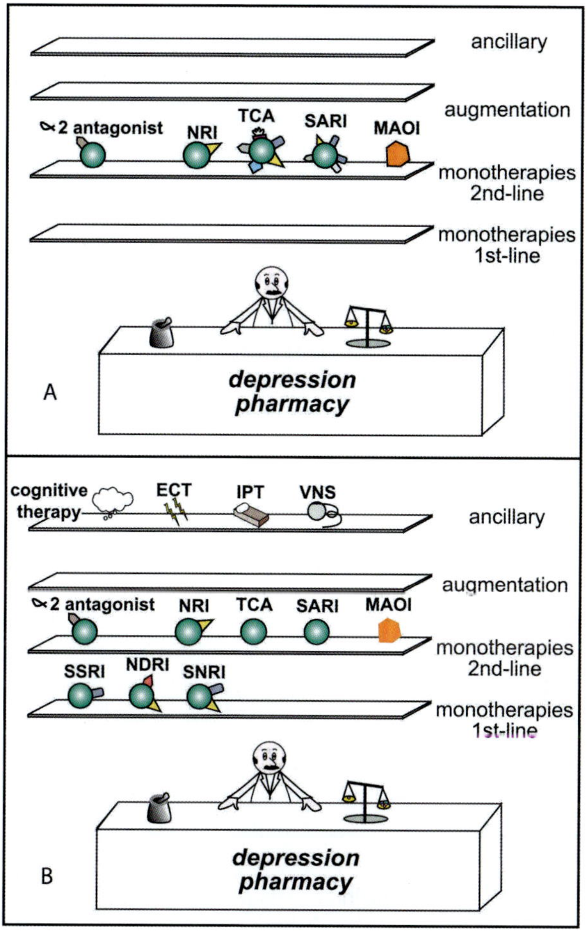

FIGURE 8.22. If a monotherapy plus augmenting agent are not successful in attaining symptom remission, a second-line monotherapy may be introduced (A). Finally, ancillary treatment options may also be recommended (B).

SSRI: selective serotonin reuptake inhibitors. NDRI: norepinephrine and dopamine reuptake inhibitors. SNRI: serotonin norepinephrine reuptake inhibitors. ECT: electroconvulsive therapy. IPT: interpersonal therapy. VNS: vagus nerve stimulation. NRI: norepinephrine reuptake inhibitors. TCA: tricyclic antidepressants. SARI: serotonin 2A antagonist/reuptake inhibitors. MAOI: monoamine oxidase inhibitors.

Following First-Line Monotherapies with Symptom-Based Antidepressant Augmentation Strategies

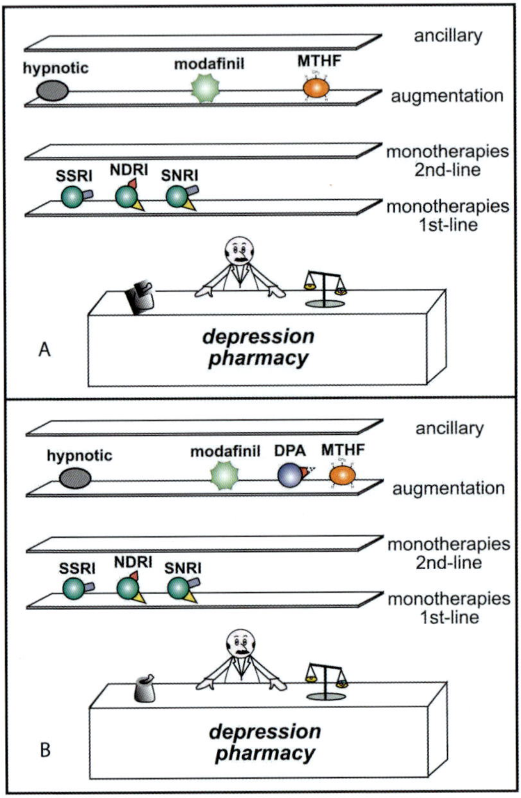

FIGURE 8.23. A symptom-based approach after failure of first-line monotherapies could be a hypnotic if residual insomnia, modafinil if residual fatigue/problems concentrating or L-methylfolate if the patient has had problems tolerating prior treatments, since this should have few if any side effects (A). If the patient is still not in remission, augmentation with an atypical antipsychotic (e.g., aripiprazole) starting at low doses may be considered (B).

SSRI: selective serotonin reuptake inhibitors. NDRI: norepinephrine and dopamine reuptake inhibitors. SNRI: serotonin norepinephrine reuptake inhibitors. DPA: dopamine partial agonists. MTHF: L-5-methyl-tetrahydrofolate.

Psychotherapy

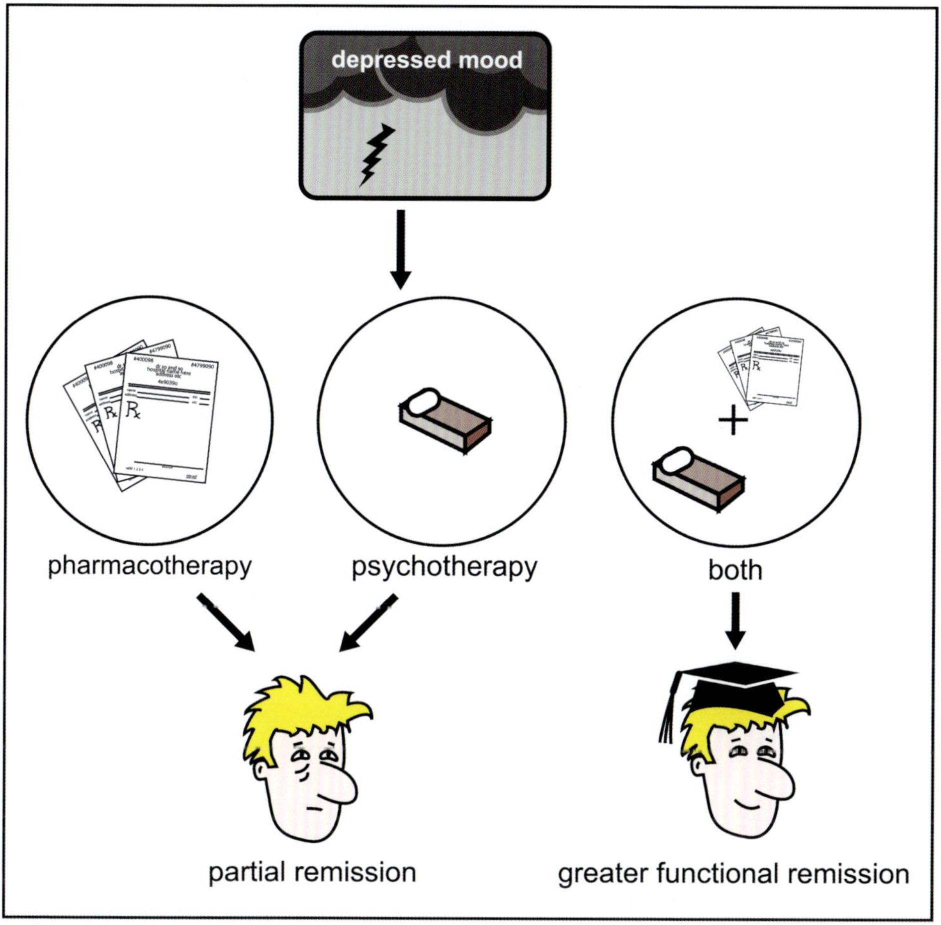

FIGURE 8.24. Psychotherapy adjunct to pharmacotherapy has been shown to improve overall quality of life in patients with major depressive disorder. Behavioral and educational therapies help improve factors such as total functioning, relationship functioning, life satisfaction, compliance with medication, and personal coping mechanisms. Psychotherapy can provide a necessary regular forum for patients to express and work through the progression of their illness and the coping mechanisms they use to overcome their limitations.

Stahl's Illustrated | Summary

- Three neurotransmitters involved in the regulation of depressive symptomatology were discussed: serotonin, norepinephrine and dopamine
- Circuits include pathways extensively traveled by 5HT, NE and DA
- Various genes are risk factors for depression
- Depression can often be treatment-resistant, resulting in the need for several different drug combinations prior to achieving response and full remission
- There are currently many classes of antidepressants available, with SSRIs, SNRIs and NDRIs most often considered first-line treatment options
- Augmentation of these first-line treatments can be selected by using a symptom-based strategy; that is, choose treatments most likely to reduce each individual patient's specific symptoms based upon the underlying neurobiological rationale for these symptoms
- Several new treatments for depression are on the horizon

Abberviations and Symbols

5HT	serotonin
A	amygdala
ACh	acetylcholine
BF	basal forebrain
CYP450	cytochrome P450 system
DA	dopamine
DAT	dopamine transporter
DBS	deep brain stimulation
DLPFC	dorsolateral prefrontal cortex
H	hippocampus
Hy	hypothalamus
NDRI	norepinephrine dopamine reuptake inhibitor
Li	lithium
MAOI	monoamine oxidase inhibitors
MTHF	l-5-methyl-tetrahydrofolate
NDDI	norepinephrine dopamine dishinhibitor
NDRI	norepinephrine dopamine reuptake inhibitor
NE	norepinephrine
NET	norepinephrine transporter
NRI	norepinephrine reuptake inhibitor
PFC	prefrontal cortex
SARI	serotonin antagonist/reuptake inhibitor
SERT	serotonin transporter
SNDI	serotonin and norepinephrine disinhibitor
SNRI	serotonin norepinephrine reuptake inhibitor
SSRI	selective serotonin reuptake inhibitor
T	thalamus
TCA	tricyclic antidepressant
TMM	trimonoamine modulator
TMS	transcranial magnetic stimulation
VMPFC	ventromedial prefrontal cortex
VNS	vagus nerve stimulation

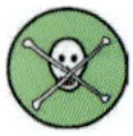	Life-threatening or Dangerous Side Effects	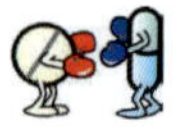	Drug Interactions
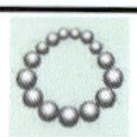	Tips and Pearls		Cardiac Impairment
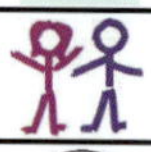	Children and Adolescents	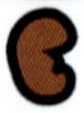	Renal Impairment
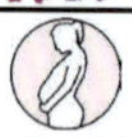	Pregnancy	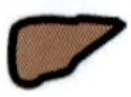	Hepatic Impairment

Stahl's Illustrated

Suggested Readings

Avery DH, Holtzheimer III PE, Fawaz W, Russo J, Neumaier J, Dunner DL, Haynor DR, Claypoole KH, Wajdik C and Roy-Byrne P. A controlled study of repetitive transcranial magnetic stimulation in medication-resistant major depression. Biol Psychiatry 2006;59(2):187–94.

Barone P, Scarzella L, Marconi R, Antonini A, Morgante L, Bracco F, Zappia M and Musch B. Pramipexole versus sertraline in the treatment of depression in Parkinson's disease. J Neurol 2006;253:601–7.

Berman RM, Marcus RN, Swanink R, McQuade RD, Carson WH, Corey-Lisle PK and Khan A. The efficacy and safety of aripiprazole as adjunctive therapy in major depressive disorder: a multicenter, randomized, double-blind, placebo-controlled study. J Clin Psychiatry 2007;68.843–853.

Cavanagh J, Patterson J, Pimlott S, Dewar D, Eersels J, Dempsey MF and Wyper D. Serotonin transporter residual availability during long-term antidepressant therapy does not differentiate responder and nonresponder unipolar patients. Biol Psychiatry 2006;59(4):301–8.

Cipriani A, Barbui C, Brambilla P, Furukawa TA, Hotopf M and Geddes JR. Are all antidepressants really the same? The case of fluoxetine: a systematic review. J Clin Psychiatry 2006;67(6):850–64.

Cipriani A, Pretty H, Hawton K and Geddes JR. Lithium in the prevention of suicidal behavior and all-cause mortality in patients with mood disorders: a systematic review of randomized trials. Am J Psychiatry 2005;162:1805–19.

Cooper Kazaz R, Apter JT, Cohen R, Karagichev L, Muhammed-Moussa S, Grupper D, Drori T, Newman ME, Sackeim HA, Glaser B and Lerer B. Combined treatment with sertraline and liothyronine in major depression: a randomized, double-blind, placebo-controlled trial. Arch Gen Psychiatry 2007;64(6):679–88.

Crossley NA and Bauer M. Acceleration and augmentation of antidepressants with lithium for depressive disorders: two meta-analyses of randomized, placebo-controlled trials. J Clin Psychiatry 2007;68(6):935–40.

DeMartinis NA, Yeung PP, Entsuah R and Manley AL. A double-blind, placebo-controlled study of the efficacy and safety of desvenlafaxine succinate in the treatment of major depressive disorder. J Clin Psychiatry 2007;68(5):677–88.

Dew MA, Whyte EM, Lenze EJ, Houck PR, Mulsant BH, Pollock BG, Stack JA, Ensasi S and Reynolds III CF. Recovery from major depression in older adults receiving augmentation of antidepressant pharmacotherapy. Am J Psychiatry 2007;164:892–9.

Dording CM, Mischoulon D, Peterson TJ, Kornbluh R, Gordon J, Nierenberg AA, Rosenbaum JE and Fava M. The pharmacologic management of SSRI-induced side effects: a survey of psychiatrists. Ann Clin Psychiatry 2002;14(3):143–7.

Emslie GJ, Yeung PP and Kunz NR. Long-term, open-label venlafaxine extended release treatment in children and adolescents with major depressive disorder. CNS Spectr 2007;12(3):223–33.

Epstein J, Pan H, Kocsis JH, Yang Y, Butler T, Chusid J, Hochberg H, Murrough J, Strohmayer E, Stern E and Silbersweig DA. Lack of ventral striatal response to positive stimuli in depressed versus normal subjects. Am J Psychiatry 2006;163(10):1784–90.

Fava M. Augmenting antidepressants with folate: a clinical perspective. Clin Psychiatry 2007;68(Suppl 10):4–7.

Fava M, Graves LM, Benazzi F, Scalia MJ, Iosifescu DV, Alpert JE and Papakostas GI. Across-sectional study of the prevalence of cognitive and physical symptoms during long-term antidepressant treatment. J Clin Psychiatry 2006;67(11):1754–8.

Frank E, Kupfer DJ, Buysse DJ, Swartz HA, Pilkonis PA, Houck PR, Rucci P, Novick DM, Grochocinski VJ and Stapf DM. Randomized trial of weekly, twice-monthly and monthly interpersonal psychotherapy as maintenance treatment for women with recurrent depression. Am J Psychiatry 2007;164:761–7.

Fu CHY, Williams SCR, Brammer MJ, Suckling J, Kim J, Cleare AJ, Walsh ND, Mitterschiffthaler MT and Andrew CM, Pich EM and Bullmore ET. Neural responses to happy facial expressions in major depression following antidepressant treatment. Am J Psychiatry 2007;164:599–607.

Gibbons RD, Hur K, Bhaumik DK and Mann JJ. The relationship between antidepressant prescription rates and rate of early adolescent suicide. Am J Psychiatry 2006;163 :1898–1904.

Goodwin FK and Jamison KR. (eds) Manic depressive illness. New York, NY: Oxford University Press; 1990.

Gould GG, Altamirano AV, Javors MA and Frazer A. A comparison of the chronic treatment effects of venlafaxine and other antidepressants on serotonin and norepinephrine transporters. Biol Psychiatry 2006;59:408–14.

Guzzetta F, Tondo L, Centorrino F and Baldessarini RJ. Lithium treatment reduces suicide risk in recurrent major depressive disorder. J Clin Psychiatry 2007;68(3):380–3.

Hedlund PB, Huitron-Resendiz S, Henriksen SJ and Sutcliffe JG. 5-HT7 receptor inhibition and inactivation induce antidepressant like behavior and sleep pattern. Biol Psychiatry 2005;58(10):831–7.

Hoyer D, Hannon JP and Martin GR. Molecular, pharmacological and functional diversity of 5-HT receptors. Pharmacol Biochem Behav 2002;71:533–54.

Keedwell PA, Andrew C, Williams SCR, Brammer MJ and Phillips ML. The neural correlates of anhedonia in major depressive disorder. Biol Psychiatry 2005;58:843–53.

Keedwell PA, Andrew C, Williams SCR, Brammer MJ and Phillips ML. A double dissociation of ventromedial prefrontal cortical responses to sad and happy stimuli in depressed and healthy individuals. Biol Psychiatry 2005;58:495–503.

Kellner CH, Knapp RG, Petrides G, Rummans TA, Husain MM, Rasmussen K, Mueller M, Bernstein HJ, O'Connor K, Smith G, Biggs M, Bailine SH, Malur C, Yim E, McClintock S and Sampson S. Continuation electroconvulsive therapy vs. pharmacotherapy for relapse prevention in major depression: a multisite study from the Consortium for Research in Electroconvulsive Therapy (CORE). Arch Gen Psychiatry 2006;63:1337–44.

Kennedy SH, Konarski JZ, Segal ZV, Lau MA, Bieling PJ, McIntyre RS and Mayberg HS. Differences in brain glucose metabolism between responders to CBT and venlafaxine in a 16-week randomized controlled trial. Am J Psychiatry 2007;164:778–88.

Kessing LV, Søndergård L, Kvist K and Andersen PK. Suicide risk in patients treated with lithium. Arch Gen Psychiatry 2005;62:860–6.

Kugaya A and Sanacora G. Beyond monoamines: glutamatergic function in mood disorders. CNS Spectr 2005;10(10):808–19.

Lemke MR, Brecht HM, Koester J and Reichmann H. Effects of the dopamine agonist pramipexole on depression, anhedonia and motor functioning in Parkinson's disease. J Neurol Sci 2006;248:266–70.

Levinson DF. The genetics of depression: a review. Biol Psychiatry 2006;60:84–92.

Marek GJ, Martin-Ruiz R, Abo A and Artigas F. The selective 5-HT2A receptor antagonist M100907 enhances antidepressant-like behavioral effects of the SSRI fluoxetine. Neuropsychopharmacology 2005;30:2205–15.

Mayberg HS. Defining the neural circuitry of depression: toward a new nosology with therapeutic implications. Biol Psychiatry 2007;61:729–30.

Mayberg HS, Lozano AM, Von V, McNeely HE, Seminowicz D, Hamani C, Schwalb JM and Kennedy SH. Deep brain stimulation for treatment-resistant depression. Neuron 2005;45:651–60.

McGrath PJ, Stewart JW, Fava M, Trivedi MH, Wisniewski SR, Nierenberg AA, Thase ME, Davis L, Biggs MM, Shores-Wilson K, Luther JF, Niederehe G, Warden D and Rush AJ. Tranylcypromine versus venlafaxine plus mirtazapine following three failed antidepressant medication trials for depression: a STAR*D report. Am J Psychiatry 2006;163:1531–41.

McMahon FJ, Buervenich S, Charney D, Lipsky R, Rush AJ, Wilson AF, Sorant AJM, Papanicolaou J, Laje G, Fava M, Trivedi MH, Wisniewski SR and Manji H. Variation in the gene encoding the serotonin 2A receptor is associated with outcome of antidepressant treatment. Am J Hum Genetics 2006;78(5):804–14.

Meyer JH, McNeely HE, Sagrati S, Boovariwala A, Martin K, Verhoeff NPLG, Wilson AA and Houle S. Elevated putamen D2 receptor binding potential in major depression with motor retardation: an [11C] raclopride positron emission tomography study. Am J Psychiatry 2006;163:1594–1602.

Michelson D, Adler LA, Amsterdam JD, Dunner DL, Nierenberg AA, Reimherr FW, Schatzberg AF, Kelsey DK and Williams DW. Addition of atomoxetine for depression incompletely responsive to sertraline: a randomized, double-blind placebo-controlled study. J Clin Psychiatry 2007;68(4):582–7.

Millan M. The role of monoamines in the actions of established and "novel" antidepressant agents: a critical review. Eur J Pharmacol 2004;500(1-3):371–384.

Mitchell ES and Neumaier JF. 5-HT6 receptors: a novel target for cognitive enhancement. Pharmacol Ther 2005;108(3):320–33.

Montgomery SA and Andersen HF. Escitalopram versus venlafaxine XR in the treatment of depression. Int J Clin Psychopharmacol 2006;21(5):297–309.

Najt P, Perez J, Sanches M, Peluso MAM, Glahn D and Soares JC. Impulsivity and bipolar disorder. Eur Neuropsychopharmacol 2006;17(5):313–320.

Nemeroff CB, Mayberg HS, Krahl SE, McNamara J, Frazer A, Henry TR, George MS, Charney DS and Brannan SK. VNS therapy in treatment-resistant depression: clinical evidence and putative neurobiological mechanisms. Neuropsychopharmacology 2006;31:1345–55.

Nierenberg AA, Keefe BR, Leslie VC, Alpert JE, Pava JA, Worthington JJ 3rd, Rosenbaum JF and Fava M. Residual symptoms in depressed patients who respond acutely to fluoxetine. J Clin Psychiatry 1999;60(4):221–5.

Nierenberg AA, Adler LA, Peselow E, Zornberg G and Rosenthal M. Trazodone for antidepressant-associated insomnia. Am J Psychiatry 1994;151(7):1069–72.

Nierenberg AA, Cole JO and Glass L. Possible trazodone potentiation of fluoxetine: a case series. J Clin Psychiatry 1992; 53(3):83–5.

Nierenberg AA, Farabaugh AH, Alpert JA, Gordon J, Worthington JJ, Rosenbaum JF and Fava M. Timing of onset of antidepressant response with fluoxetine treatment. Am J Psychiatry 2000;157:1423–8.

Nierenberg AA, Fava M, Trivedi MH, Wisniewski SR, Thase ME, McGrath PJ, Alpert JE, Warden D, Luther JF, Niederehe G, Lebowitz B, Shores-Wilson K and Rush AJ. A comparison of lithium and t3 augmentation following two failed medication treatments for depression: a STAR*D report. Am J Psychiatry 2006;163:1519–30.

Nierenberg AA, Ostacher MJ, Calabrese JR, Ketter TA, Marangell LB, Miklowitz DJ, Miyahara S, Bauer MS, Thase ME, Wisniewski SR and Sachs GS. Treatment-resistant bipolar depression: a STEP-BD equipoise randomized effectiveness trial of antidepressant augmentation with lamotrigine, inositol, or risperidone. Am J Psychiatry 2006;163:210–6.

Oquendo MA, Currier D and Mann JJ. Prospective studies of suicidal behavior in major depressive and bipolar disorders: what is the evidence for predictive risk factors? Acta Psychiatr Scand 2006;114(3):151–8.

Pace TWW, Mletzko TC, Alagbe O, Musselman DL, Nemeroff CB, Miller AH and Heim CM. Increased stress-induced inflammatory responses in male patients with major depression and increased early life stress. Am J Psychiatry 2006;163(9):1630–3.

Papakostas GI and Fava M. A meta-analysis of clinical trials comparing milnacipran, a serotonin-norepinephrine reuptake inhibitor, with a selective serotonin reuptake inhibitor for the treatment of major depressive disorder. Eur Neuropsychopharmacology 2007;17:32–6.

Papakostas GI, Shelton RC, Smith J and Fava M. Augmentation of antidepressants with atypical antipsychotic medications for treatment-resistant major depressive disorder: a meta-analysis. J Clin Psychiatry 2007;68(6):826–31.

Pae CU, Peindl K, Hooper-Wood C, Mannelli P and Ciccone P. A randomized, double-blind, placebo-controlled trial of augmentation with an extended release formulation of methylphenidate in outpatients with treatment-resistant depression. J Clin Psychopharmacol 2006;26:653–6.

Pitchot W, Hansenne M, Pinto E, Reggers J, Fuchs S and Ansseau M. 5-hydroxytryptamine 1A receptors, major depression and suicidal behavior. Biol Psychiatry 2005;58(11):854–8.

Rapaport MH, Gharabawi GM, Canuso CM, Mahmoud RA, Keller MB, Bossie CA, Turkoz I, Lasser RA, Loescher A, Bouhours P, Dunbar F and Nemeroff CB. Effects of risperidone augmentation in patients with treatment-resistant depression: results of open-label treatment followed by double-blind continuation. Neuropsychopharmacology 2006;31:2505–13.

Roberson-Nay R, McClure EB, Monk CS, Nelson EE, Guyer AE, Fromm SJ, Charney DS, Leibenluft E, Blair J, Ernst M and Pine DS. Increased amygdala activity during successful memory encoding in adolescent major depressive disorder: an fMRI study. Biol Psychiatry 2006; 60(9):966–973.

Robertson B, Wang L, Diaz MT, Aiello M, Gersing K, Beyer J, Mukundan Jr S, M Carthy G and Doraiswamy PM. Effect of bupropion extended release on negative emotion processing in major depressive disorder: a pilot functional magnetic resonance imaging study. J Clin Psychiatry 2007;68(2):261–7.

Rush AJ, Trivedi MH, Wisniewski SR, Stewart JW, Nierenberg AA, Thase ME, Ritz L, Biggs MM, Warden D, Luther JF, Shores-Wilson K, Niederehe G and Fava M. (2006) Bupropion-SR, sertraline, or venlafaxine XR after failure of SSRIs for depression. N Engl J Med 354; 12, 1231–1242.

Sanacora G, Kendell SF, Levin Y, Simen AA, Fenton LR, Coric V and Krystal JH. Preliminary evidence of riluzole efficacy in antidepressant-treated patients with residual depressive symptoms. Biol Psychiatry 2007;61(6):822–5.

Schaefer HS, Putnam KM, Benca RM and Davidson RJ. Event-related functional magnetic resonance imaging measures of neural activity to positive social stimuli in pre-and post-treatment depression. Biol Psychiatry 2006;60(9):974–86.

Schechter LE, Ring RH, Beyer CE, Hughes ZA, Khawaja X, Malberg JE and Rosenzweig-Lipson S. Innovative approaches for the development of antidepressant drugs: current and future strategies. NeuroRx 2005;2(4):590–611.

Schramm E, van Calker D, Dykierek P, Lieb K, Kech S, Zobel I, Leonhart R and Berger M. An intensive treatment program of interpersonal psychotherapy plus pharmacotherapy for depressed inpatients: acute and long-term results. Am J Psychiatry 2007;164:768– 77.

Shang Y, Gibbs MA, Marek GJ, Stiger T, Burstein AH, Marek K, Seibyl JP and Rogers JF. Displacement of serotonin and dopamine transporters by venlafaxine extended release capsule at steady state. J Clin Psychopharmacol 2007;27(1):71–5.

Shelton RC, Haman KL, Rapaport MH, Kiev A, Smith WT, Hirschfeld RMA, Lydiard RB, Zajecka JM and Dunner DL. A randomized, double-blind, active control study of sertraline versus venlafaxine XR in major depressive disorder. J Clin Psychiatry 2006;67(11):1674–81.

Siegle GJ, Thompson W, Carter CS, Steinhauer SR and Thase ME. Increased amygdala and decreased dorsolateral prefrontal BOL responses in unipolar depression: related and independent features. Biol Psychiatry 2007;61:198–209.

Skidmore FM, Rodriguez RL, Fernandez HH, Goodman WK, Foote KD and Okun MS. Lessons learned in deep brain stimulation for movement and neuropsychiatric disorders. CNS Spectr 2006;11(7):521–37.

Takano A, Suzuki K, Kosaka J, Ota M, Nozaki S, Ikoma Y, Tanada S and Suhara T. A dose-finding study of duloxetine based on serotonin transporter occupancy. Psychopharmacology 2005;185:395–9.

Thase ME. The failure of evidence-based medicine to guide treatment of antidepressant nonresponders. J Clin Psychiatry 2006;67(12):1833–55.

Thase ME, Clayton AH, Haight BR, Thompson AH, Modell JG and Johnston JA. A double-blind comparison between bupropion XL and venlafaxine XR. J Clin Psychopharmacol 2006;25(5):482–8.

Thase ME, Corya SA, Osuntokun O, Case M, Henley DB, Sanger TM, Watson SB and Dube S. A randomized, double-blind comparison of olanzapine/fluoxetine combination, olanzapine, and fluoxetine in treatment-resistant major depressive disorder. J Clin Psychiatry 2007;68(2):224–36.

Thase ME, Friedman ES, Biggs MM, Wisniewski SR, Trivedi MH, Luther JF, Fava M, Nierenberg AA, McGrath PJ, Warden D, Niederehe G, Hollon SD and Rush AJ. Cognitive therapy versus medication in augmentation and switch strategies as second-step treatments: a STAR*D report. Am J Psychiatry 2007;164:739–52.

Trivedi MH, Fava M, Wisniewski SR, Thase ME, Quitkin F, Warden D, Ritz L, Nierenberg AA, Lebowitz BD, Biggs MM, Luther JF, Shores-Wilson K and Rush AJ. Medication augmentation after the failure of SSRIs for depression. N Engl J Med 2006;354:1243–52.

Trivedi MH, Rush AJ, Wisniewski SR, Nierenberg AA, Warden D, Ritz L, Norquist G, Howland RH, Lebowitz B, McGrath PJ, Shores-Wilson K, Biggs MM, Balasubramani GK and Fava M. Evaluation of outcomes with citalopram for depression using measurement based care in STAR*D: implications for clinical practice. Am J Psychiatry 2006;163:28–40.

Valenstein M, McCarthy JF, Austin KL, Greden JF, Young EA and Blow FC. What happened to lithium? Antidepressant augmentation in clinical settings. Am Psychiatry 2006;163:1219–25.

Vanover KE, Weiner DM, Makhay M, Veinbergs I, Gardell LR, Lameh J, Del Tredici AL, Piu F, Schiffer HH, Ott TR, Burstein ES, Uldam AK, Thygesen MB, Schlienger N, Andersson CM, Son TY, Harvey SC, Powell SB, Geyer MA, Tolf BR, Brann MR and Davis RE. Pharmacological and behavioral profile of ACP-103, a novel 5-HT2A receptor inverse agonist. J Pharmacol Exp Ther 2006;317:910–8.

Wagner KD, Kowtch RA, Emslie GJ, Findling RL, Wilens TE, McCague K, D'Souza J, Wamil A, Lehman RB, Berv D and Linden D. A double-blind, randomized, placebo-controlled trial of oxcarbazepine in the treatment of bipolar disorder in children and adolescents. Am J Psychiatry 2006;163:1179–86.

Wisniewski SR, Fava M, Trivedi MH, Thase ME, Warden D, Niederehe G, Friedman ES, Biggs MM, Sackeim HA, Shores-Wilson K, McGrath PJ, Laori PW, Miyahara S Suggested Reading and Rush AJ. Acceptability of second step treatments to depressed outpatients: a STAR* D report. Am J Psychiatry 2007;164:753–60.

Zarate CA, Singh JB, Carlson PJ, Brutsche NE, Ameli R, Luckenbaugh DA, Charney DS and Manji HK. A randomized trial of an N-methyl-D-aspartate antagonist in treatment resistant major depression. Arch Gen Psychiatry 2006;63:856–64.

Zarate CA, Singh JB, Quiroz JA, DeJesus G, Denicoff KK, Luckenbaugh DA, Manji HK and Charney DS. A double-blind, placebo-controlled study of memantine in the treatment of major depression. Am J Psychiatry 2006;163:153–5.

Zimmerman M, McGlinchey JB, Posternak MA, Friedman M, Attiullah N and Boerescu D. How should remission from depression be defined? The depressed patient's perspective. Am J Psychiatry 2006;163:148–50.

Stahl's Illustrated | Index

Stahl's Illustrated

Posttest

CME credit has expired for this activity (2/28/15). You are welcome and encouraged to complete the posttest for your personal enrichment, but will not be able to receive credit nor print a certificate for this activity.

Posttest Study Guide

PLEASE NOTE: The posttest can only be submitted online. *The posttest questions have been provided below solely as a study tool to prepare for your online submission.* ***Faxed/mailed copies of the posttest cannot be processed*** *and will be returned to the sender. If you do not have access to a computer, contact NEI customer service at 888-535-5600. There is a fee for the posttest (waived for NEI Members).*

1. After four successive antidepressant treatments over the course of one year, what percentage of patients will achieve remission?

   A. 33%
   B. 40%
   C. 50%
   D. 67%

2. What is the difference between the monoamine hypothesis of depression and the neurotransmitter receptor hypothesis?

   A. Antidepressants block the reuptake pump/Antidepressants block the post-synaptic receptors
   B. Monoamines are increased due to blockade of reuptake pump/Monoamines are increased leading to down-regulation of receptors
   C. Monoamines are increased in the presynaptic neuron/Monoamines are increased in the postsynaptic neuron
   D. Antidepressant administration results in disinhibition of monoamines/Antidepressant administration results in inhibition of monoamines

3. SSRIs may have which of the following secondary pharmacologic properties?

   A. Alpha 2 antagonism
   B. Inhibition of nitric oxide synthetase (NOS)
   C. Norepinephrine and dopamine disinhibitor actions (NDDI)
   D. A and B
   E. B and C
   F. A and C

4. What area of the brain has decreased levels of dopamine transporters?

A. Striatum
B. Basal forebrain
C. Thalamus
D. Prefrontal cortex

5. SNRIs may increase which of the following in the prefrontal cortex?

A. Serotonin
B. Dopamine
C. Norepinephrine
D. A and C
E. B and C
F. A, B and C

6. Which postsynaptic serotonin receptor is most affected by the increase of serotonin release due to mirtazapine blockade of alpha 2 heteroreceptors?

A. 5HT1A
B. 5HT2A
C. 5HT2C
D. 5HT3

7. Individuals taking a monoamine oxidase inhibitor should completely avoid all foods containing tyramine.

A. True
B. False

8. Which of the following is true about depression and reproductive hormones?

A. Depression is linked to estrogen levels in women across the life span
B. Depression is linked to testosterone levels in men across the life span
C. A and B
D. Neither A nor B

9. What is unique to the mechanism of action of serotonin antagonist/reuptake inhibitors (SARIs)?

A. Serotonin is excitatory at 5HT1A receptors and inhibitory at 5HT2A receptors
B. 5HT2A agonism does not affect 5HT1A antagonism
C. Blockade of 5HT2A receptors contributes to inhibitory potentiation of stimulating 5HT1A receptors
D. Stimulation of 5HT2A receptors leads to decreased 5HT

10. Which of the following pharmacologic properties is true of all tricyclic antidepressants?

A. Block reuptake of both serotonin and dopamine
B. Agonists at alpha 1 adrenergic receptors
C. Block voltage-sensitive calcium channels
D. Antagonists at muscarinic cholinergic receptors

11. Which antipsychotic was recently approved for use as a unipolar depression add-on?

A. Olanzapine
B. Quetiapine
C. Aripiprazole
D. Risperidone

12. According to the symptom-based algorithm for antidepressant selection, which of the following would best be utilized for treatment of apathy in depression?

A. Fluoxetine + olanzapine
B. Escitalopram + eszopiclone
C. Bupropion + modafinil
D. Fluoxetine + trazodone

Online Posttest

You can complete the posttest and activity evaluation at **www.neiglobal.com/CME** (under "Book"). If you do not have access to a computer, contact customer service at 888-535-5600. There is a fee for the posttest (waived for NEI members).